INSIGHT

Out of Mind

John D. Day

PAGE PUBLISHING, INC.
New York, NY

First originally published by Page Publishing, Inc. 2017

ISBN 978-1-64027-141-8 (Paperback)
ISBN 978-1-64027-142-5 (Digital)

Printed in the United States of America

INTRODUCTION

Kale called from a nearby motel, "Hey man! You told me to call you if things got worse! Well…, it's not good!"

"Why? What's up?" I ask. "What's happening?"

"I don't want to talk about it on the phone," he answers, "Can you come here?"

"Why? What the hell is goin on? Where are you?"

"I'm at that sixth street motel, room 12… They're starting to come through the TV now! What the hell am I gonna do?"

"Hold on!" I respond. "I'll be there in a few minutes!"

I arrive at his room and knock on the door. He cautiously peaks through the curtains, opens the door, steps out to take a suspicious look around, then motions for me to come in. Contrary to his usual cocky display of self-confidence, he looks exhausted and uneasy. He sits down on the end of the bed. Staring at the TV, he takes a gulp of his beer. Calmly, I ask what the problem is. He hesitates. With the hand that's gripping the beer, he points at the TV and through a casual, yet affirming voice he declares, "The things I used to hear in my head are now coming through the TV and through the radio in my car."

Aware of his recent condition, I point at his beer and say, "Do you think you should be drinkin?"

"Ah," he shrugs, "seems to keep 'em quiet."

As I pause in search of a proper response, we are both reminded of our familiarity during this brief, uncomfortable silence. Recognizing my hesitation and before I could speak, he looks up to say, "Look, man. This is not my imagination! Either these people are really fuckin with me now or I am completely losing my mind. I think it's time we go find out if I'm really fucking crazy!" He makes eye contact once again and with that unyielding stare I've known most of my life, he asks, "You up for it?"

For the first time in my life, I am seriously afraid for my friend. He's been hearing voices...

NOTE TO READER

I too am sick. I now find myself in sunny Arizona, where it has been raining for three days, and I can't help but think I am somehow responsible. Maybe the ominous cloud that has been hovering over my life has decided to follow me here. But I know this too shall pass—it's Arizona. I arrived last week in my toy hauler, along with my Harley, my dirt bike, and my cat (had no choice). I still owe the bank on two of the three, and the cat was free. I'm in search of sunshine. I left the sanctity and security of my small-town habitat in order to escape the dark, cold winters of the upper Midwest, where my depression is accentuated by relentless snowstorms and frigid temperatures that confine you indoors. Well, there is that, and hangovers. I may also be here trying to prove the most recently introduced type of depression actually exists, called SAD (seasonal affective disorder). Its obvious claim is that the lack of sunshine has a direct effect on the brain. I will likely have a more accurate depiction as time passes.

Being a true creature of habit, the small-town lifestyle I acquired years ago during winters consists of ice fishing, heavy drinking, and way too much time to think; there isn't much else to do. I decided that in order to finish this story, I have to escape to a warmer climate and find a reasonable form of isolation in order to 'get right'. Don't get me wrong, I love my friends back home, and I have the tendency to party with them as much as I am allowed at forty-four years old, but my hangovers tend to bring on an onset of guilt, culpability, and outright depression. I'm not just tired and run-down after a night of drinking—I become a stagnant wretch! This is something that I've dealt with most of my life, and it would seem that if I stayed sober, this problem would solve itself.

I am now and will be sober as I write this. In the past, I've frequently gone months without any outside form of medicine, drug, or alcohol, yet I still awake to an indescribable feeling of loss and dejection. This has gone on as long as I can remember, and the lack of finding a solution multiplies this frustration. I have survived by family, music, poetry, 'forced' exercise, and laughter with friends. I feel good today, and it may have to do with isolation, eating right, exercise, or just working at something I like to do, or simply, sunshine.

I am and have always considered myself to be the human guinea pig of life, and as much as I've tried to cure myself with alcohol, it has yet to happen. And I have also come to realize while writing this story, that at times it may sound like, but is not intended to be, a written pity party. I hate sensing that someone feels sorry for me. Don't. The characters I speak of would say the same. Your sympathy is not required. I simply wrote this because I made a promise to my friend.

Although psychiatry seems to have evolved to now focus on more of a chemical path to a solution, they always believe in counseling, which can often bring bad memories to the forefront. I suspect you will point fingers and likely experience animosity, possibly toward undeserving people, such as family members that may or may not deserve any blame. I ask you not to. It's my opinion that mental illnesses occur likely through no one's fault, maybe just through one's chemical makeup, because of the way our brain causes us to think, and not the way some psychologists would often have us believe—that the way we were raised has caused our lives to be dysfunctional. We are not the result of mistakes.

The acknowledgement of this theory may be necessary, and conversations with those involved in our pasts may have to take place. But to me, it seems rude and unjust to make another feel bad just so we can feel good. Is that how we are to feel better? I don't completely agree. Somehow, it is like blaming the original source, a long-forgotten relative, likely one that has been dead for hundreds of years now, in hope of finding the rightful source of abuse, neglect, and bad parenting. It is like an attempt to chase down the guilty party, to appoint blame to a parent, who will rightly blame their own parents, because this is always handed down from generation to generation. Was it my great-great-grandfather? Did he abuse or neglect his sons and daughters? If so, isn't it possible he did so accidently, while working hard, struggling to survive? I find no comfort in cursing him. So I offer family members a preempted apology if I cause readers to think poorly of everyone's parenting skills. I will still give you the truth knowing you will judge to your liking. You have that right.

I believe that the genes I have inherited, this chemical makeup of my mind, is not the accumulation of years of child abuse or neglect. The proof of this is in the remedy: a pill. Personally, I've found that by taking the right one, oblivious to the purpose, can make me create a smile, go to work, be kind and patient with my son, and forget that I was ever sick and never look back. I just haven't found one that can last, and I don't enjoy the side effects. I am currently taking only natural vitamins.

I am a huge fan of the written word. I love the places my mind goes (when allowed) while enjoying a good book. As far as writing a book, it feels good to be able to speak, or write, without interruption, knowing that what I say cannot be taken out of context because it's still in the context. That feels liberating. I'm picturing sitting down with a good friend who has all the time in the world to listen without judgment. Since I can't see you, I won't gauge your reactions and alter my story, as I know I have sometimes done during conversation, in order to suit your facial expressions so as to comfort and please you. I won't have to increase the speed of my story when I observe you losing interest. I do require you to keep an open mind so I can feel free to tell the truth. You will be updated on my personal struggle throughout the story.

My journal has been my friend since 1994. I will share it with you while I do this, but it's mine again afterward. This should be an easy read for you. I have the vocabulary of your neighborhood electrician. Feel free to buy this book for a friend who says, "I haven't read a book since high school!"

CHAPTER 1

Small Town

Nowhere to Hide:

It began within me and I haven't outgrown.
Depression is real. It exists on its own.
Are others born lucky? Free from the dark?
Do they live on the outside? Do they get the
    'walk in the park'?
I'm jealous of healthy. I envy the sane.
They drift forward with ease and here I remain.
So I'll sit in this sadness that is myself;
Praying tomorrow will bring something else.
It comes and it goes with a selfish stride.
Three days of freedom, but there's nowhere to
    hide.

—"Nowhere to Hide"

(Actual current daily journal entry. Written while writing.)

1/5/14. I have no reason to feel ill today. Yesterday, I felt ill for no reason. I don't mean sick like having the flu or sick as in wishing for my death. I felt like I often do; empty. Where thoughts enter, but never stay. I tend to blame this on alcohol, as I should. On New Year's Eve, six days ago, I had a glass of wine before the bar, 8 beers, two shots, five captain cokes, and an 8 ounce bottle of champagne. (Kept the receipt.) Happy New Year! All of this was done in the course of 6 to 7 hours. I did eat during this so the hangover was expected, yet not too extreme. It lingered for a couple days and that's normal. I recognize that would seem like a lot of alcohol, but if you knew where I came from…

I've never considered myself a true alcoholic. I remember a therapist once called me a problem drinker. That I can understand. I don't think of myself as an alcoholic because I can stop. I will find my proper balance while I continue this story. There is no other way for me to do this.

—January 5, 2014

I have to describe where it is that I do come from: small-town Midwest, USA—small as in a population of two hundred, small as in nine-man football, small as in "My mom is the mayor," small as in "I see Joe got a new truck, must be nice." I had no control over arriving here at two years old, and why I haven't left is still an unanswered question. I'm sure it has a psychological answer.

Time here seems to stand still. You can truly leave for a year and nothing will change and you can be brought up to speed with the locals within an hour of conversation. But to say that I don't like it here would be a lie. I've lived in a few other places in the Midwest, but I've always come back. Whether I'm physically here or not, it will always be home.

I joke, but the people here do spend much of their time in other people's business by no fault of their own. It seems unavoidable—there's not enough of your own business. On any given day, the local farmers, philosophers, and intellectuals can be found at the local café exchanging monologues or just discussing last night's game. I consider the majority of the community to be moderate Christians. It is and remains a safe place to raise children. The neighborhood watch is always in full force, but a parent can also become complacent. Knowing there are adult eyes everywhere, you tend to forget to keep the parent-child lines of communication open. As a child, you love the freedom, but as a parent, it is too easy to assume all is well. I know this because my son spent much of his childhood here as well.

If this town has any hindrances, one, at least for me, would be the freedom of expression. I like to think outside the box. This makes it difficult to express your opinions openly. Back then, I, like my father, was not one for confrontation. The act of telling some-one face-to-face what you truly think of them might be the cause for many uncomfortable moments at the local gas station or grocery store, although most of the community is very tolerable, like fam-ily—only annoying if you see too much of them. We are kind here, but I was often too passive. I still am.

Withholding these truths from sensitive acquaintances as an adult is minor compared to what a child feels. Peer pressure is in full force with every child anywhere. Feeling and being different from the majority can be cause for humiliation, particularly in a small town where it's difficult to find others who share your same ideals. I obvi-ously found my sanctity with my friends from the north side of town.

This small-town's scenic view is flat. It consists of snowdrifts in the winter and corn and beans in the summer. Farming is why it exists. We're located almost a hundred miles from an actual city and two hundred miles from a major city. Geographically, they call it the rolling plains, with the exaggeration on the *rolling*. *Plain* is the best description. It's possible for winters here to last six months, and if we don't receive snow, you end up looking at baron-plowed fields with an occasional dirt drift—not too inspirational. (Then again, as a child, your vision seems as short as your attention span, so I didn't complain then. I didn't know better.) The wind is a constant, and the proof is in the recent placement of wind towers. The sun seems absent most of the winter and appears to cause the locals to become a little restless. It definitely has this effect on me.

It seems that every source of entertainment revolves around alcohol and bars. (There might be other forms of recreation, but I have yet to know what they are.) They do create snowmobile trails, if weather permits, and many lakes are within reach for ice fishing. Otherwise, the entertainment has to take place indoors. There is always a dart league or pool league to join. Bands are not as common now, but there is the ever-present karaoke. The area is speckled with similar small towns, all within ten to twenty miles away that partake in the same activities. Everywhere you go, someone you know is always having a birthday or anniversary or getting married or divorced, so it's easy to find reason to celebrate.

As a child, I believed this town to be much larger. I walked two blocks to school every morning across the lawns I mowed for cash in the summertime. I rode my bicycle everywhere. My parents both worked, so I had a handful of friends with whom I'd spend most of my time as they loved to hang out at our home. We had hideouts we called forts in abandoned buildings or shelterbelts (tree lines), where we would sneak off to smoke cigarettes, build or destroy things, and daydream. I was a very happy child.

I am the youngest of three. My brother Josh is three years older and my sister Sharlene, five. Early on, my father worked at various local jobs—school custodian, bus driver, and he once owned the grocery store, until he became a manager at the local gas station / hardware store. My mother also worked locally as a secretary/bookkeeper.

Although my father's job at the local gas station was taxing and would prove to be very cruel and unrewarding as he neared retirement, he tried to spend as much time as he could with us while we were young. I feel he deeply regretted the twenty four years he dedicated to his job. When he could find the time, he would often take our family and whoever wanted to join, fishing at the nearby lakes. He'd also hit baseballs to my brother and me after work. We played Little League baseball, football in the backyard, and basketball on a netless rim in the neighbor's dirt alley. (Xbox had yet to be invented.) I acquired a minibike at the age of nine. I was spoiled in this regard.

I worked. I mowed lawns and delivered newspapers, but I didn't truly know what money meant at this age, as I believe most children shouldn't. I would be told by my mother what it was we could afford and I seemed to accept that. I understood we were not wealthy. When my mother proceeded to pour a bowl of cereal in front of my friend, I stated, "Hey, I thought you said we were supposed to quit feeding the neighbors." (Mom likes to remind me of that from time to time.)

In a child's eyes, the separation of classes in my south-side neighborhood could be determined by what type of cereal you possessed. If you had Lucky Charms in the cupboard, you were rich! If we did happen to have it, it was a special treat and gone in a day. My parents worked hard. They provided. If something of material was missing in my life, I was as much unaware of it then as I am now.

I recall receiving my first concussion of many at this young age—running as fast as I could on the playground and sliding across the ice. During a collision with another kid, the back of my head landed solid on the ice. It would be several seconds before I was brought back to consciousness. Fearing punishment, it was agreed to be kept a secret, but only for a short time. Dazed, I came in from recess and sat down in class. Feeling nauseous, I immediately excused myself to the bathroom and was met by my father, the custodian at the time, in the hallway. He noticed I was pale and asked what was wrong. Before I could answer, I vomited on the floor. I was sent home for the day. Had the ice cracked, I would have been given some relief of impact. I remember them telling me specifically that it didn't.

(Concussions are a prominent cause of depression.)

CHAPTER 2

My Second Family

I didn't know it was depression. I thought I was
    doing wrong.
I spent so much time inside my mind; the spon-
    taneity of life was gone.
Now it's a slippery surface that I walk upon and I
    pretend that I won't fall.
But the sadness comes like rain pouring down
And I forget that I was happy, at all.

I was eleven years old in the fall of 1981. I was returning from my paper route on my minibike when I first remember meeting Kale. He and my brother, Josh, had the trunk of my parents' car open in the driveway, admiring the contents. In the way teenagers disregard their younger siblings, there would be no formal introductions. Kale already knew who I was—his new friend's little brother. I approached to see what looked to be dead animals. As I gazed upon the pile of carcasses of raccoons and muskrats, Kale rubs my head and states, "Bet there's over a hundred bucks in there, Johnny! Wanna help skin 'em?"

Sheepishly, I reply, "Ah ... no thanks!"

Kale was wearing a faded, possibly bleached jean jacket, dirty jeans soaked with grease and blood, and work boots that have traveled way too many miles for a teenager. He was also ripped! At this time, he stood about five feet eight inches, with blond hair and piercing blue eyes, and was thin yet had a very muscular physique, wiry. Veins protruded from his arms when called for. His skin was dark from too many hours in the sun. His hands were calloused and scarred from manual labor. His nose looked to have permanent swelling between the nostrils from having at least once been broken. He was fourteen years old but older than he looked. He was the prototypical 'greaser', and I was amazed.

At the time, I had no idea Kale was currently dating my sister. At eleven years old, my sixteen-year-old sister's dating habits were not a priority, and girls were still 'stupid' at my age. I was informed by some of my classmates that a new family had moved to our small school as some of my same age but further advanced male friends took an interest in Kale's younger sister, Tanya. My brother had also been hanging with some new friends from just outside of town as he had recently obtained a driver's license (a permit was allowed at fourteen in our state). Therefore, he was rarely in my presence. I didn't mind. I was busy. I had a paper route, lawns to mow, a minibike to ride, and no desire to grow up anytime soon.

Josh and Kale had become friends through JV football, with Josh reporting that Kale was one of the roughest players on the team. It seemed he had convinced my brother to drive him around to help him check his traps. My father had taken us pheasant hunting and fishing, but trapping was new to my brother and me. It seemed deep-rooted to Kale.

I believe it was sometime between the fall of '81 and the spring of '82 that the Taylor family moved to town. I would see Kale with my sister on occasion at my home, and through him, I would eventually meet the rest of the family—Tanya, Daniel, Steve, and their mother, Joan.

Joan was a single mother with a steady job. This left their home open often so it also became a safe haven from adults. Their house was a larger square, two story home built around the same time as mine and only a block away from where I currently reside. Linoleum floors, slightly worn and used furniture, it would be clean only until the next time the boys messed it up. And if you happened to be there during cleaning, you helped. (Being unkempt and over a hundred years old, this old house was recently demolished. Mine is likely next.)

"Friends are relatives you make for yourself"
(Eustache Descamps).

Inside their home was a lifestyle to which I was unaccustomed. There seemed to be no rules governing your behavior when Joan was absent. Steve and Daniel were in charge as they were already the size of full-grown men. If they approved of your conduct, you seem to have been safe from the outside world. You could cuss, smoke, drink (not me yet), argue, and experience life in reality, taking in all the emotions that expressing one's self causes. I'm not avoiding anyone or anything at home, but for reasons unbeknown, I would come to spend almost as much time at this house as my own. They would become like family. At times it seemed hectic to me, but it was real.

Although it never happened in my presence, the brothers fought. For whatever the reason, it was not to be denied. Joan tried her best to keep control of her home, and at my young age, I preferred to be there more often in her presence than not. In times of chaos, she was composed and could instantly freeze everyone and get their complete attention by hollering "All right!" at the appropriate moment. I took pleasure in watching her larger, unruly sons cower to her when she laid down the law. They seemed to fear no one but their mother. She was and still is the strongest woman I know.

Joan Taylor is a remarkable woman, beautiful inside and out. At this time, I believe she was in her late thirties (none of my business) and had seen her share of hard times. She was also slender and strong yet had an inner strength beyond human understanding. She listened like no other and always defended me from her sons when their ribbing got out of hand. With her on your side, you couldn't lose. She was and has always been the one to turn to. She was a rock—no, she was stronger. She was a diamond.

Joan's mother also lived in the home but was rarely seen. She stayed in her room on the second floor most of the time and appeared to be antisocial. I would rarely see her, and as rude and uncouth as children could be, we would jokingly warn one another to stay away from 'crazy' grandma.

I would mow the Taylors' lawn in the summer as this was often my excuse to spend time there. Steve was already out of school. He was very mechanically inclined and would be occupied in the yard, working on his beloved Dodge, wearing his 'wife-beater' shirt and greasy, rim-bent baseball cap. He had reddish-blonde hair with dark roots, shoulder-length, and always donned some type of facial hair. I would often convince him to help do the trim work with the push mower while I drove my father's riding mower. In winter, when the snow was deep, I would persuade Steve to drive me around on his snowmobile to deliver papers, primarily in blizzard conditions. He'd only ask for gas money. Steve was more quiet, passive, and reserved than his brothers. He was not adverse to mocking and teasing someone like me, but he was unassuming, and I felt a sense of calm in his presence, always have. He was the man of the house.

Scoob, my good friend and classmate, and I once tested Steve's mistakenly passive demeanor and his strength. It was wintertime, with over a foot of snow on the ground. Scoob and I were likely riding high due to an altercation a week earlier. We had a confrontation with my brother while playing basketball at a neighbor's snowplowed driveway. Scoob had recently been witness to several poundings from my brother, Josh, inflicted upon me, likely due to my recently acquired ability to hold my own on the court. Apparently, the violent fouls I was receiving from my brother were more than Scoob could tolerate. I was used to it but also tired of it. In the heat of the game, he decided to assist me, and it soon escalated into a fight. Together, we gave Josh a fairly good beatdown and left him bleeding and lying in a snowbank. I felt a hint of guilt and a forewarned sense of repercussion while walking away, but Scoob assured me that he had it coming and told me to tell Josh that if he did retaliate, we'd do it again.

While at Joan' house, with this newfound confidence, Scoob and I bragged about our scuffle to Steve. He expressed to us that Josh wasn't quite a man yet and that he was likely going to retaliate when the time was right. We didn't seem too concerned with Steve's insight. We told him that together, we could kick the shit out of most full grown men. Steve opposed our notion as he attempted to inform us about the difference between boy strength and man strength.

Now Steve was almost twenty years old. He's about six feet tall and well-built. He and his brothers all had a broad back and this certain type of build to them that, through the years, I had learned to recognize early. It was not that they didn't look strong; they were just surprisingly stronger than they looked. This 'man strength' discussion increased in intensity, at least from Scoob's point of view. I knew where it was leading, and I was hesitant. Steve had likely had enough of our boasting, so without showing any emotion, including anger, he convinced us to step outside and give him our best shot.

I tried to first establish ground rules. "Are we punching faces, choking, kicking, wrestling, you know? What's the limit?" Steve instructed us to choose whatever means necessary to win. He confidently assured us he'd be fine. With Steve standing on the snow-swept sidewalk and Scoob and myself a few feet away, Steve announced while giggling, "Well, I'm ready!" Seconds later, Scoob dived for his legs, and I swung an overhand right somewhere toward Steve's head. I can't explain what happened next because I honestly don't know. What I do remember a few seconds later was being held facedown in the snow, struggling for air. I could hear a similar muffled scream next to me. Steve calmly asked if we were done as we made some sound resembling "Yes." He helped us up and dusted us off while we reentered the house. I somehow sustained a bloody nose in the melee, so while leaning over the sink, Steve helped to clean me up while wearing a restrained smile. It deemed a necessary humiliation—so many lessons to learn.

Daniel, the middle son, was somewhat of a jock. He was the tallest of the boys, listed at 6'3" on the basketball roster. He was also involved with track, football, and cross-country. He was the athletic, tall, dark, and handsome guy. He bore the same physique as his brothers but wasn't as rugged looking. Daniel had a soothing, deep, Johnny Cash-like voice. It appeared he was also the voice of reason in most situations at the Taylor home. I would hear about him from the admiring, ogling girls in my class before I remember meeting him.

I can remember a girl I would later date sharing her story of how she broke her pelvis during a fall while practicing for cheerleading. Instead of strapping her on a gurney, Daniel happened by and carried her out to the ambulance. She said that was the best part of the ordeal. I would watch her recite her story to others with such awe and wonderment in her expression.

Although Daniel was somewhat intimidating and very capable, he did not appear to be violent. Silently admired by his family and openly admired by the rest of us, he was more outgoing and sociable than his brothers. Although he would harass my friends and me often, he never seemed to mean any harm. He was more empathetic than others his age. You would feel a slight more important just being in his presence as his confidence seemed contagious and was never mistaken as arrogance. To an impressionable kid unconsciously searching for a role model, he was the one!

In the summer of 1983, I found myself wearing braces and glasses. I was not happy about it. I was not happy about many things. I must be a late bloomer because my friends and classmates were growing around me and I was still a small kid. I checked my armpits daily, waiting for a miracle. At my second home, I was frequently terrorized for my shortcomings, although I was learning how to give and take shit. The brothers liked to tease Tanya and me about our relationship because they saw me there often and assumed she was the reason. Maybe she was.

Tanya was tall for her age, definitely taller than me at this time. She was slender and strong like her brothers. She was very outspoken and was undeniably a tomboy. My friends found her attractive, but due to the amount of time I had spent in their home, I seemed to have put her in the friend/sister category. If there was something more, I was unaware of it. I was often at their home because girls were becoming a factor now, and Tanya's classmates, one year younger than me, were commonly visiting. (In small-town schools, you have to act fast. Class size is around twenty to thirty kids. If your friend saw her first, you're out of luck.)

Many lessons were learned in the Taylors' north-side home. From the simplest of tasks, like how to light your smoke with a toaster, how to heat the kitchen by using the stove, how to lock your bedroom door with a knife, how to make the grossest-looking but best-tasting scrambled eggs for a party of six, how to make coffee, how to burn garbage, how to change a flat, how to start your car by shorting out the starter and how to push start a four-speed if that didn't work, how to pick a lock, how to wrestle, how to box, how to use nunchakus and throwing stars, how to modify an antenna with aluminum foil, how to make tinsel using beer tabs, how to play cards, how to shotgun a beer, how to make up your own words to songs and to the English language in general. And to the more meaningful things, how to respect your elders, how to take school and sports seriously, how to provoke then comfort your friends in times of stress (to get it out and move on?), how to listen and how to know when to walk away, how to laugh hysterically at yourself and others, and how to cry.

I experienced these similar sentiments at home, but they were not commonly displayed. My family seemed more cautious and reserved. Early on in my life, on Sundays, our family would go to church together, eat together, and visit relatives. As soon as my sister was nearing graduation and Josh and I were accumulating more friends and becoming involved in more social activities, sports, etc., we didn't seem to do a lot together. I don't think my parents ever missed one of our games throughout high school, but after my sister left home, our dining room table rarely saw us all together, apart from holidays. I can still hear my father yelling from the stairway on Sunday mornings, telling us he was leaving for church soon, but we'd hide under our covers until he gave up. I guess I was choosing to learn my spirituality by taking a much-less-traveled path.

Greaser

My sister, Sharlene, had recently graduated high school and was attending a technical college nearby. Kale was still dating her, minus a few breakups in between. He was still a constant source of ribbing, directed mostly toward my brother and me, possibly instigated by unavoidable relationship issues with my sister. He based much of his accusations in reference to his all-time favorite movie, *The Outsiders*. It had just been released. (It's a story based on the differences among well-to-do kids, the south-side socials, or socs, pronounced [so-shez], from the suburbs; and the poor kids, the greasers, from broken homes. Kale had also read the book. Although exaggerated, it seemed to match the criteria.) My family lived on the south side of town, my parents were still married, we lived in a new home, and our vehicles were not new but ran without constant maintenance. We could afford new clothes, shoes, etc. While Kale claimed when he started football, he had to wear work boots.

Kale was from the north side of town, his parents were divorced, his home needed paint and repairs, and most of his clothes he swore he had to buy himself with money he made trapping, working for area farmers, and building grain bins in the summer. Much sooner than most, Kale knew the value of money. He had valid justifications, yet his razzing seemed to be given and taken lightly. He was just a prideful young man, likely somewhat envious of our lifestyle and our relationship with our father, reminding my brother and me from time to time that our lives were, in fact, different.

Kale first humorously demonstrated his reasoning one day while we were standing in Joan's kitchen making peanut butter sandwiches. He watched me slowly spreading Skippy nice and neat to the corners of my slice of bread. He pointed and exclaimed, "See, look how you so-shez eat!"

Frozen, I replied, "What the hell are you talking about? How do you do it?"

He replied in a dainty tone, "You 'so-shez' have to make sure your peanut butter is spread so perfect." He quickly dipped the knife to the bottom of the jar and excavated all he could and grabbed a slice of bread, which lay flat on the palm of his hand. Without hesitation, he swiped the knife across the bread and folded it in half, squeezing all the peanut butter off the knife and onto his now-half sandwich. He paused to look at me then shoved almost all of it in his mouth. With his mouth stuffed full, he managed the words "Ya know? Just eat the son of a bitch!" We both almost choked with laughter.

I would come to see things in a different light every time I was in Kale's presence. Even as a young teenager, he was always expanding my mind. I was drawn to his abnormal sense of humor. I gave some question as to why I liked to be around someone who was, admittedly, sometimes abrasive and rude. It may have been because he had no fear of being rude. Maybe it was because he had what I lacked: guts. Maybe it was because he didn't seem to need many friends, and I tended to need all of them. Maybe it was the openness he forcibly created, the direction he caused me to think, the bold statements, and the respect he commanded by displaying the fact that he was original and real. And I was not. Maybe it was because even though his actions were unpredictable and unruly, his overall behavior was consistent. Or maybe it was just because he made me laugh. Like it or not, through no fault of anyone or anything and without our knowledge or awareness, but as sure as the sun will rise, I was unwittingly becoming the protégé, and Kale was my mentor.

What likely cemented Kale's hero eminence in my mind was what I witnessed in the summer of '83. Kale, Josh, and I were at a nearby lake. They were likely scoping out areas to set traps for the upcoming season. Josh and Kale had a casual six-pack between them as I was likely not allowed to drink. At thirteen, I was happy just to be along. We would meet a couple of teenagers who arrived on an ATV. They were from another school but seemed to share mutual friends. They were both drinking, but one of the two seemed to be on a mission. After about an hour, this fifteen-year-old kid walked away from the group with the half gallon of whiskey and began to chug it like water. By the time we noticed and stopped him, he had consumed more than a human body should ever be required to endure. Several minutes later, he managed to stagger away from the group and fell flat on his face on the gravel road. Now barely coherent, bleeding out both nostrils, we helped him to his feet.

We shared time holding him up and trying to walk with him as the sun went down. His friend said it would be impossible to bring him home on the ATV and had no intention of returning him to his parents in this condition. He asked if we could take him in our car while he retrieved a different vehicle to meet up with us back in town. He was placed him in the backseat with me.

We arrive at our vacant elementary-school parking lot as I heard gurgling sounds and erratic breathing coming from him in the backseat. I told Josh something was seriously wrong. He quickly parked the car. Kale turned to look in the back and immediately stepped out. He pulled our new, helpless friend from the backseat, and we stood him up against the car. His face had now lost color, and his body had gone limp. Wiping off more of the dried blood that had accumulated around his nose and mouth, Kale yelled, "He's fuckin chokin' on something! Hold him up!" As Josh and I propped him up against the car, Kale forced the guy's head back and stuck his fingers down his throat. The kid tried to gag. Frustrated, and on his second or third attempt, Kale pulled out a dark-red ball of blood the size and shape of a mouse and threw it down on the road with a smack! Immediately, the kid sprung to life and began vomiting. After which, he inhaled deep breaths. He was choking on his own blood! A few minutes later, Kale directed us to walk him around the parking lot. He began speaking after a while as his friend eventually arrived and escorted him home.

I have since reminded this person about this night as he has never had any recollection of it, but I don't know if he completely understands how close he was to death. But then again, he no longer drinks, so maybe he does understand. This scene was rarely spoken of again between Kale and me as he often downplayed drama or heroics, but I wouldn't forget.

CHAPTER 3

Daniel

> Had a great day! Why? Could be due to the following: Reliving the past and enjoying it, reaffirming the answer to the never ending question; who am I? Or the feeling that this is possibly starting to read like a book, believing I can do something with my life, or maybe exercise and sunshine, or vitamins, or proper sleep, or sobriety. It's 7pm. Happiness is fading with the thought of what's next. Tired, was up early. Tomorrow: Not looking forward to what I have next to write. Ttyl. Not depressed, tho.
>
> —January 9, 2014, daily journal (unedited)

At thirteen, I was still a slave to my brother, and we'd begin our days before school by scrambling and yelling at each other as we both had trouble with mornings. He seemed to be the only one of his friends who had 'wheels', and my job was to warm up the car, head to the Taylors' (north side), and roust the brothers for their ride to school. A bus was always available, but they were way too cool to be seen riding it. (Our school system is a consolidation of three neighboring small towns, and our high school is located about ten miles south of ours.)

Between the three of them—Daniel, Kale, and Josh—and sometimes a straggler, they often managed to scrounge enough for gas. That, and my father, being the most unselfish man the world has ever seen, would allow us to charge gas to him at the local station where he now worked. Daniel seemed to always be the first to be ready, and on occasion, if we had time while we waited, he'd direct me to the local store to start his day with chocolate milk and a 7Up. During which time he'd give me advice on every topic I had in question. Sports and girls were often our main subjects. I valued his attention.

I didn't always like having to do the early-morning slave work, but it would mean I'd be in the company of, whom I believed to be, the most popular kids in school. As an eighth grader, to be hanging with my brother and the Taylors would prove to raise my status with the rest of the school. I was still somewhat of an awkward kid, barely over 5 feet tall, 110 pounds and sporting new glasses and braces. I could use all the help I could get! Just to walk through the halls and get a noogie or a punch in the arm from one of these guys would establish my rank among my friends. It also helped to keep other bullies at bay. It seemed that no one in their right mind was going to risk even a conversation with Daniel or Kale about why they chose to trouble me. *They* could rough you up, but you couldn't, just like family.

Through the word on the street, Kale and Daniel's badass reputation had already been firmly cemented in the minds of other teenagers. Daniel seemed to establish his dominance with his straightforward approach to conflicts, but mostly with his tone and choice of words. Daniel was not a violent teenager. Clashes were unavoidable in high school, yet he had a way of approaching conflicts with humor and reasoning. And the more you got to know him, you would realize how levelheaded and kind he was to others. If he did become offended, he was likely defending someone else. He always looked out for the underdog.

Kale, on the other hand, was not as forgiving. At this age, if threatened, he frequently chose to swing first and ask questions later. There was a fire burning inside him early on, and it was safe to assume that he must have suffered several beatdowns growing up, assumingly by the hands of his alcoholic father. He was also likely retaliating for once having been smaller and weaker. Even the older, larger kids knew to draw the line with him. Although the odds might be in their favor, they knew they would likely be risking their life. And Daniel would be next in line.

Kale frequently worked out on a makeshift punching bag, lifted weights, and studied Bruce Lee. He would often show me a new move he learned or created meant to quickly dismantle an opponent. He appreciated the art of fighting, but it seemed it was a violent world he lived in, even at this young age.

Displaying such a defensive personality may have kept Kale from having an abundance of close friends, though he didn't seem to mind. He had his brothers, several cousins, a group of older friends (fellow bin builders), and me and Josh to befriend. The girls in school also seemed to admire him. They thought of him as a rebel, the mis-understood hero portrayed in most movies.

In the fall of '83, the uncomfortable braces that I sported had to be adjusted often at the orthodontist in our nearby 'college' town. Our high school and football field was on the way to my appoint-ments, so my mother had me ride with Josh to early-morning foot-ball practices before these appointments. I was playing junior high football but was still in question of playing the game at the next level. As an eighth grader, I was still patiently waiting to physically mature. Through watching the older players in practice, I was becoming a huge fan.

Their team would have a fairly successful football season that year. Daniel was chosen homecoming king, and justly so. He was very popular, well-liked by the 'so-shez' and the 'greasers', and an above-average football and basketball player. He excelled in track and cross-country as he held the long jump record for many years. He was highly admired, had at least one beautiful girlfriend, and was an excellent role model. He definitely fit the profile. I didn't know anyone who didn't like him. He would graduate the following spring and began working road construction nearby.

1984

> The formative years of high school would prove to contain lessons that should be reserved for adults.

One year later, it was a typical Friday afternoon in October—game day. Upon returning home from school, I organized my football gear, ate my usual pregame meal, and meditated in front of the TV- a ritual; all things I learned from watching my brother. He was now a senior. I was an undersized freshman. I had yet to be on the field during a close varsity game, but it couldn't hurt to imitate those who have. Waiting for Josh for my signal to head to the north side and retrieve Kale and Dave, our other greaser friend, and Josh's classmate, I lost patience and took a ride on my ATV. I ventured by Taylors' home. I knocked once and walked right in like I always did, only to find no one around. I returned home and relayed this information to Josh. He uttered a half-hearted response like he knew they might not be there so I went about my business. He told me to call their home right before we leave to see if they wanted a ride to the game.

I called. Daniel answered with enthusiasm, "Yeah?" I was surprised by his voice. I didn't know he was back from working on the road.

"Hey. Daniel?" I asked.

He recognized me. "Hey, Johnny!"

"Am I supposed to pick up Kale and Dave?" I asked.

"They're still washin' uniforms from last week! Believe that? Naw, we're gonna take Kale's new car. Heard you might get some playin' time tonight?"

"Yeah, second string back is out tonight, so I could at least be returning kicks," I replied.

"Cool. Maybe I'll get to see ya play?"

Feeling more nervous about the realization of playing, "Yeah" was all I could muster.

Before hanging up, he paused. "Hey, good luck tonight, Johnny!"

Josh and I met up with the bus and informed the coach of the situation as he was aware that Dave and Kale normally rode with us. The coach waited several minutes but decided we had to leave without them. I believe he was secretly hoping they'd at least drive themselves to the game since they were very important players. He announced to the team, "We might be shorthanded tonight, so you underclassmen, be ready to play!" They were the last words an under-sized running back like me wanted to hear. It meant that in the process of moving players around, I would likely see some action. I gave only a brief thought to just what the hell Kale and Dave were doing. They didn't seem to care too much about tardiness for school, but to be late for a football game? I told myself they were just running late and would drive themselves to the away game's field. There would be repercussion from the coach for doing so, but he wouldn't dare stop Kale and Dave from playing. I let my thoughts settle with that scenario and returned to thinking about football. "Just don't fumble" was my mantra.

It was a beautiful night for football—stars shining and little wind, cold but tolerable. I had yet to play. Sometime early in the second half, there was an abrupt interruption to the game. Our sideline and our fans were faced opposite the entrance to the complex. The game was abruptly halted as a policeman and a couple of adults, I couldn't see who, walked straight across the field toward our fans instead of going around. They were looking for Dave's parents. Word got out that there had been a car accident. It was quickly assumed that Dave had been injured.

This was the only information given. Roaming the sidelines while the game ensued, I asked some of the staff for more details, but very little was forthcoming. I was young and naive, so when told to focus on the game, I obeyed. For the life of me, I can't recall if I played or if we won. It seemed miniscule compared to what I remember next.

Cold, dirty, and exhausted, the team filed into the bus. Standard postgame conversation among the players was in session when the coach entered and asked for our attention as he told us to sit down. The only light in the bus was from the field lights outside and the exiting cars in the parking lot. Head down, he struggled for words. "There has been a terrible car accident. Kale and Dave have been injured but are in stable condition. Their injuries are serious but don't appear to be life-threatening. Kale's brother Daniel didn't make it. He passed away at the scene." After a long silent pause, he finished, "Don't lollygag in the showers. Let's get home so we can find out just what happened." I looked for my brother's face, but he was seated several rows behind me.

Located a few blocks from the field, we arrived at the opposing team's locker room. I sat on the bench. There was no sound other than running water and background whispers from the staff about usual postgame procedures. Being young and living in a small environment, this would be my and many others' first personal brush with death. There was no one in the room who didn't know who Daniel was, at least by being last year's homecoming king and football standout. My brother, who always seemed to openly display appropriate emotions, had his head down with tears in his eyes and was slowing packing his clothes. I was stoical. It would be days, weeks, before I emotionally acknowledged this tragedy. My thoughts were with my brother. Daniel and Josh were tight. I thought about Joan, Steve, and Tanya, and the severity of Kale's and Dave's injuries.

We arrived at our high school. I silently hung around my brother. I never knew his plans; I just stayed within sight so I could manage a ride home. We walked the half block to the local pool hall, the usual stop after a game. Emotions ran high. In the light from the streetlights, I could hear and see people standing around their vehicles, quietly exchanging information and rumors, crying and hugging. Some were handling it aggressively. In the distance, I could hear a lot of 'what-the-fucks' and 'who-the-fucks'?! We received sketchy information as to where it happened, what car they were driving, how fast they were going, and who was driving. My brother and his girlfriend were a short distance away from the rest of the crowd. Josh was stooped between two parked cars in the darkness and was crying. He was devastated. His girlfriend was ineffectively attempting to comfort him. She had trouble understanding the depth of his emotions. She appreciated what the word *family* meant; she just didn't know how far ours reached.

In the morning, on the way to the hospital to visit Kale and Dave, we investigated the scene of the accident. It took place two miles short of their destination. This blacktop road had been seal-coated with pea rock over the summer. It had been worn to almost its original form in the paths of the wheels of traffic, but there were always loose rocks in the middle and on the sides and shoulders that took longer to settle. The skid marks began at the intersection where there was a slight hump noticed only at high speeds; it was slight, but it was enough to extend your shocks while driving the speed limit. Approximately a hundred yards south, there were two approaches for driveways to two opposite farm homes. The skid marks began right after this slight hump and veered across traffic, just beyond the second approach. There was a line of full-grown trees to the east, fifty to sixty feet tall, protruding along a fence line separating the yard from the ditch of the highway. Josh and I walked around in silence, taking it all in. I looked up from the ditch to see broken branches, missing bark, and large gouges in several trees about fifteen feet up from where I stood. I had a vivid imagination. I thought to myself, less than fifteen hours ago, this was where their car was. The sight had obviously been cleared, but among the shattered glass and frag-mented parts in the grass surrounding the area, we happened across a small rubber toy alligator. It was often placed throughout the Taylor home and in our vehicles. We would place lit cigarettes in its mouth and squeeze to get a laugh. My brother smiled briefly and put it in his pocket. (I believe it was later placed in Daniel's casket.)

By this time, it was understood that Kale's car was a 1970 Dodge Demon, bright orange, powerful, and very fast. I hadn't seen much of Kale prior to this and was unaware he had purchased a new car after his summer of building bins. He had only owned it a few weeks. It had been said that they were likely traveling in excess of a hundred miles per hour. A witness had met them a couple of miles before the accident and confirmed that Kale was driving but kept this informa-tion a secret until the cops quit asking. Kale and Dave couldn't recall any of the evening or how the accident happened. Because of the slight hump and the loose gravel, the car likely skidded toward the left at the intersection due to the high speed they were traveling. It apparently became airborne when it left the road as the marks in the trees were well above the road's elevation. Daniel was likely ejected upon impact with the trees.

According to those who first arrived on the scene, Kale and Dave were also ejected from the car and were lying on the road several yards from each other and what was left of the car. The motor itself was said to be over a hundred feet from the point of impact. Dave was bleeding heavily as he had severed an artery under his arm. He had cuts from broken glass all over his body. When found, he was said to be yelling, "Let off the brake! Let off the brake!" Kale had broken his wrist and his arm and was also bleeding from several places. He was said to be begging the paramedics and others to tell him if his brother was okay. They knew the severity of Daniel's head injuries, so their professional response was "We don't yet. We're working on him." It was believed he died at the scene.

At the hospital, Kale and Dave were both now in stable condition and allowed to have guests. There were several friends from school there to see them. Still in their hospital gowns, Kale approached me and nodded for me to follow him. We walked down the hall toward an exit. A nurse stopped us, and before she spoke, Kale said, "We just want to step out for a smoke. Please?" She gave us a look of disgust and walked away. Outside, not knowing what to say, I asked questions regarding his injuries, like how many stitches he had and what was broken. He answered halfheartedly.

Halfway through the smoke, his tone changed, and with a puzzled look, he leaned in and whispered, "Hey, was I driving?" I believe he had already been told the answer but wanted to hear from someone he trusted. I nodded. His puzzled look turned to dejection as I believe this was his only hope of avoiding responsibility for his brother's death. I would've loved to tell him Daniel was driving. He looked off in the distance, took the last drag of his smoke, and flicked it. It would be years before we spoke intimately of this again.

The funeral was held in a recently constructed church on the outskirts of town, several blocks away from the high school. It was obviously a packed house. Prince's song "When Doves Cry" was just released and played often on the radio. Dave and Kale were still sporting bandages and casts. I sat behind the family. I cried for the first time in public since I was a toddler. We buried Daniel at the graveyard east of town. His gravesite would be visited way too many times by the young and innocent and by those who were expected to move on with their lives.

Through the power of the resilience of youth, we pressed on. The following weeks were somewhat of a blur as time went on. I would often hear my brother talking in his sleep, sometimes crying in his sleep. I never did ask him about it. I also had reoccurring dreams about Daniel. In my dream, I would be driving my brother's car by the scene of the accident, the same highway we traveled to and from school every day. Daniel would be walking along the side of the road. I'd stop, pick him up, and say, "What the hell, man? You're supposed to be dead!"

"Yeah, crazy shit, huh?" he'd reply. He'd then tell me to take him to town so we could find the boys. I had this dream on several occasions. I'm not going to pretend to know what it means, if anything.

November 1984

Kale returned to school with a newfound focus. He was held back in first grade, likely due to his family's late return from Alaska when he was just six. He was my brother's age but was considered a junior in high school. After taking some classes with seniors and others with the junior class, he managed to complete the necessary requirements and graduate with my brother's senior class, one year ahead of schedule.

Graduation day finally came in the spring of '85 for Josh and Kale. The senior annual was dedicated to Daniel. There was a poem next to his picture by an unknown author. It read,

> The people were shocked on the day of his death.
> As the story was passed, the town caught its
> breath.

Who are you kidding? It must be a lie!
He was too young, too vital to die!
The next morning the sun arose over the land
God pushed away the night with a turn of his
hand.
The birds began singing to welcome the day.
And most of the sadness was slipping away.
But the loss is imbedded so deep in our minds
That we can't leave his memory completely
behind.
Enough still remains in our hearts like a stone—
To remind us that we have lost one of our own.

I may be reaching, but I captured my last conversation with Daniel, the phone call, for personal reasons that are, obviously now, a little less personal—a very simple exchange of words that I would come to cherish. Besides being our final conversation, I think back to how self-absorbed and apathetic toward a younger generation I myself was when I was nineteen, a year removed from high school. With the excitement of after-school life just beginning, Daniel took the time to remember and acknowledge that a brother of his friend Josh, a lowly little freshman like me, was likely to be experiencing his first action in a varsity football game. He remembered. I'm proud of the fact he was even aware of this, and then to tell me he'd get to see me play still amazes me. For my lack of further articulation, let me just say that this truly explains who he was and how I will remember him.

I can't help but think how different things would have been had this never happened, how I wouldn't likely be writing this story. And trying to honor a man's life with just a few pages will always seem inadequate. Although I only knew him for a short period of time, I am certain I would have continued to know him well had he lived.

CHAPTER 4

Johnny

Az. Had to do some electrical work to aid in paying my lot rent yesterday. Felt a little off. On a scale from 1 to 10. 1 being happy, 10 being the stagnant wretch. It was about a 4. No clues as to why. Maybe I'm allergic to electrical work. But today seems okay. Depends on writing. My son seems happy back home. The sun is shining, birds are chirping. If you wonder why I keep a record of all of this; I'm hoping that if I ever end up in the shrink's office again, he can determine a pattern. Therefore, hand me the proper meds and I'll save myself some money 'getting to know him.' I realize it's okay to have an off day; everyone does. I still believe that one day in the future, I won't fear the next.

—January 15, 2014, daily
journal (unedited)

Wounds of the Day:

Words of wisdom, derived from the soul.
An artful expression, harmony's flow.
I'm just a poet, often lonely and sad.
You call this a gift, but I wish I never had.
I'd rather be simple, as it seems so free;

Opening doors, believing just to see.
An unappealing sadness follows me close;
Repelling the world, I hate more than most.
Inviting what's wrong, an unfriendly ghost,
A pity-party for all, and I am the host.
If luck is an attraction, alone I will stay;
Spitting the blood from the wounds of the day.

The summer of '85 saw Kale building bins. His older brother, Steve, was married and living in the same town as our high school and working for a cable TV company. My recently graduated brother dabbled in construction, painted houses, and delivered pizzas in our nearby college town. Kale was often gone, but I was still a frequent guest at the Taylor home. I was dating one of Tanya's close friends.

I was fifteen. I was experiencing my first love, and it was just like the Brady Bunch episode with Bobby's first kiss—skyrockets! All things sad were temporarily forgotten. I began to understand the words to love songs. We were likely a year or two behind the music scene here in the boonies, so Journey, Chicago, and the Outfield were still frequently played on the radio. I listened to Ratt, Foreigner, and Kiss when in the presence of others.

I had convinced my wonderful father to trade our ATV for a dual-purpose two-stroke motorcycle. I spent much of my time riding this motorcycle (often pushing it), playing basketball, and visiting my girlfriend at her family's home. Like any fifteen-year-old male, my mind was preoccupied with her due to high levels of testosterone. Schoolwork and all productive aspects took a backseat to thoughts of basketball and my girlfriend. I finally began to wish I was older.

Around this time, our family owned a 'Vette, a beautiful yellow two-door '79 Chevette—four-cylinder, four-speed, very fun to drive, and could achieve forty miles per gallon. It had already been abused by my brother and his friends before me. We slid across the hood and through the windows like the Duke Boys whenever we fled the scene. While en route to the lake, Kale fired a bottle rocket out the passenger window, only to have it travel over the car and back through Josh's driver's side window and into the backseat with Scoob and me.

We tried to stuff it out, but it blew up under our hands. Laughter ensued. The ashtray dangled from having once been blown up by a firecracker. All four wheels had left the ground on a few occasions.

We all owned certain scars on this poor vehicle. Kale was responsible for a rear window, which had to be replaced after he reportedly kicked it out. One story has it that he was sleeping in the back and suddenly awakened by a friend (when disturbed, he was known to wake up kicking and swinging). Others have it that he and my sister were having relationship issues while she was away at school and he acted out while drunk in a fit of rage. After asking Kale and all involved, only the 'Vette seemed to know the truth. Either way, he took responsibility for it and paid my father for the new window. (Kale always paid his debts.) I often had to have my girlfriend help to push start this car when the starter went out and I was hesitant to bring up yet another financial problem to my father. It was used to teach many drivers how to operate a manual clutch. As it often is for teenagers, this car was also the beginning of my freedom.

I was now the last one in my family still in high school. It was finally all about me. I would experiment with girls, dates, relationships, booze, cars, fights, keg parties, pot, pierced ears, graffiti, stolen merchandise, and broken laws such as underage consumptions, open container, exhibition driving, and more. I really didn't think I was a bad kid, but wow, once you write it all down … Well, I believe I was a good kid, just a people pleaser. I gave my grandma a kiss if called for, watched *Little House on the Prairie* after school, did my chores for my father, split wood, and mowed the lawn, and I was well-liked by my girlfriend's parents. I believe I was just spontaneously propelled to please and entertain those around me. If someone wanted to raise hell, well, I was always game. I can't blame myself or anyone for this. I may have been unconsciously influenced by a few older classmen, but I wasn't misinformed about the laws. I was trying to be cool and well-liked, and when you're young, naive, healthy, and involved in everyone's life, you end up at the wrong place at the wrong time much of the time. I was a teenager finding my own way. You know, just like all teenagers, I was lost and enjoying it.

Kale was on the road most of this time, and I would rarely see him. I could use his advice. I happened to be pushing my motorcycle down the highway about a half a mile from home one Saturday afternoon when I came to meet Rachel. She and Tanya stopped by in Joan's pickup to ask if I needed a ride. Tanya introduced Rachel as Kale's girlfriend. She was mysteriously pretty. She was small, Hispanic or Cuban (I still don't know; I only saw her a few times), and quite bold as she stated, "Aw, this is Johnny? He's cute!" Shying away, I told them I'd get my bike running and catch up with them later at their home. I don't recall if I did.

I would come to hear that Kale and Rachel had a son together that fall and named him Daniel, after Kale's brother. They seemed to be getting along fairly well at the time, but I can't recall much of anyone else's life at this time. I was currently quite selfish and apathetic toward my friends.

School was now tasking. I fretted over keeping my grades well enough to remain in sports. The football coach was the algebra teacher, and luckily, he was very generous. I lacked the certain focus in classes that didn't interest me. I understand that I'm not stupid; I just didn't seem to care. I seemed more concerned with what the girls were wearing, what the cooks were serving for lunch, and if the coach was going to run us tonight. I realized I now have the basics— reading, writing, and arithmetic—and I did fairly well in English and grammar. The rest seemed a waste of my time. It's my opinion that the most important thing they can teach you in high school is the desire to learn something after high school; if desire can be taught.

Basketball kept me out of trouble. Like any sport in high school, we couldn't play if your grades weren't good enough, if we've been charged with any crime involving alcohol, or if we were caught smoking or out past curfew. During basketball season, we just didn't drink. We were heavily influenced by our older siblings and friends, who would enforce this law personally. My curfew was pushed to the limit several times, but it was becoming apparent that there was too much at stake. Our coach made that perfectly clear to all of us—well, at least he did to me, as we were beginning to believe in big things as the seasons continued.

In football, we had several standouts, but overall, our team sucked. We were small. After losing a couple of games, we were mathematically out of the playoff picture. I loved the game. The problem was, I was undersized, and I basically spent three out of four quarters with a pounding headache. No one was checked for concussions back then, but knowing what I know now about the headaches, nausea, dizziness, and memory loss, I recognize I had several. (This is something I've always been drawn to when self-diagnosing depression. But it truly does me no favor now to know why.)

In the off-season, I partied. My dad sold the 'Vette to a friend of mine. I then drove a Ford Escort for a while until I upgraded to a '79 Mercury Capri: a small two-door, red with black trim, four-bolt aluminum rims, 302 V8, four-speed, and the very necessary stereo. I was happy.

Drinking and driving was a regular thing back then, and as wrong as it is, we all did our share of it. As a teen, your car is your mobile safe zone from parents. Occasionally raising hell, we would come to learn from our experienced elders to just putt around on the gravel roads surrounding our towns to avoid drawing attention. We had nick-names which were handed down from older classmen for our secret secluded hideouts; usually a gravel pit or low-maintenance road, where we'd meet up with our friends—'Badlands', 'Beer Dump road', and 'Hollywood', to name a few.

I was learning slowly. I learned humility through the power of unreturned affection during breakups with my girlfriend. It was likely when I discovered poetry. It's truly when you discover many things—what the actual song lyrics are, how to empathize, and how to create self-inflicted torture through vivid imagination and through your analytical and creative mind. At the time, I didn't believe it to be an onset of depression. I didn't ask. It seemed that no one around me really believed in depression. If they did, it wasn't openly discussed. It's not something you bring up at this age. Besides, I had reasons to feel sad sometimes.

Depression or not, this would cause me to become someone who, unintentionally, seemed to be making up for lost time during my brief monogamy. I unwittingly became more aggressive toward chasing random girls and didn't seem to want to keep a girlfriend. I began to take advantage of the younger girls' infatuations with older jocks. I remember how the girls in my class admired my brother, Josh, and Daniel and Kale. I enjoyed this positive attention. Who doesn't? But I took this to an extreme. By no means intentional and showing little self-respect, I was basically becoming a male slut. And there would eventually be consequences.

Underestimate much?

One evening that fall, I was scheduled for a rendezvous with one of my new girlfriends. I ran into Kale at the local bar. We hadn't seen each other in a while, and I was glad to sit down next to him for a visit. We first exchanged small talk of my recent football games and his work. He began to inform me about his son, Daniel, and that he and Rachel were having issues, though he seemed fairly optimistic. During our conversation, we noticed tensions were rising in the bar. Our mutual friend Dave, Dave's brother, and another friend were arguing over a game of pool with some very large strangers. (I learned later that they were once heavyweight wrestlers from a nearby college.)

Kale at this age was about 5 feet 10 inches, 180 pounds at the most. Being completely sober due to football season and training rules, I remember overhearing their conversation among the unfamiliar group. They were contemplating a violent retaliation as I recall one of them pointing and telling the others to be wary of certain individuals in the opposing group of my greaser friends. He also mentioned how he wasn't worried about the little fucker, Kale, sitting at the end of the bar.

Tempers ultimately flared across this ego-filled room. The owner somehow managed to kick everyone outside into the street, where the fighting ensued. I believe they were evenly matched man per man, with at least two fights happening simultaneously. (To offer my assistance would have been considered suicide, and I make no apologies in my admittance of it. Some of these guys were pushing three hundred pounds!) I proceeded to find a comfortable spot on the sidewalk a few yards away to witness the melee.

With both throwing a few swings, the paired-up couples would usually go to the ground within seconds. It soon became less interesting as all seemed to end up tiring from wrestling, with my friends on the bottom. They had taken somewhat of a beating before Kale intervened and separated one group. Walking away, one of the strangers flung a backhand at Kale and caught him in the face. It would be the only punch he would receive. He quickly squared up, with Kale calling him out to the street. He took his position on the street and fired a quick combination, landing a left and a right, and then he paused. Sensing it was just the beginning of a beating, the stranger turned his head and walked back to the sidewalk. Kale let him go. Kale then noticed one of our enraged friends attempting to retrieve a rifle from his car. He immediately stole it from his hands, and while chewing his ass, he locked it back in the car.

Just when I thought it was over, the shortest, yet heaviest of the group of wrestlers began to boast of their accomplishment with somewhat of swagger. Tired of the talk, Kale approached and jabbed him in the face. Again, aware of the tight corners in between the cars, Kale then lured him onto the street. With a small crowd now in attendance, he proceeded to land lightning-fast jab after jab while circling around like a prize fighter working on a heavy bag. The combinations were so quick I had trouble determining whether or not they were thrown. The sight from behind—the way his opponent's head continued to jerk backward and the intermittent view of his bloody, toothless mouth, were the only certainty.

This fight continued long enough that between them and the crowd watching, the traffic that usually traveled through the main street / highway of my small town had now proceeded to back up and reroute. Oblivious to the traffic, they were not going to stop. The beating came to a conclusion when the much-larger man fell forward and managed to bring Kale to the ground. With Kale now on his back and his opponent's face in his chest (full guard), he continued to punch from this position, often pausing to ask him if he was done. Exhausted and bleeding, the man finally submitted.

The owner of the bar where the fighting began then proceeded to bring out two cases of beer and place them on the sidewalk. "Here, stop this bullshit and drink some free beer!" he yelled.

When the two stood up, you could see the blood coming from the stranger's mouth as you notice several teeth missing from his smile. With all of them now sitting a few feet apart and surprisingly cordial on the sidewalk, exhausted and drinking their free beer, the guy with missing teeth, still spitting blood, exclaimed, "Fuck, I wasss sthupossed to go to my parenth's Thankthssgiving thissss weekend!" A wiseass from the crowd commented, "I bet if you ask Kale nicely, he'll give you back your teeth." It was truly a remarkable display of speed and technique over size and strength. It was representative of the mixed martial arts that you see today. Other than one man's trip to a dentist, it ended much better than expected. I completely forgot about my plans to meet the girl.

I would learn through Tanya that Kale's relationship with Rachel had become unstable. He continued working on the road, returning home on occasion, and though I still loved to party when training rules didn't apply, our age difference was more of an issue. I was becoming more self-absorbed. I don't mean self-absorbed like I'm focused on schoolwork or future plans. I was busy being cool and playing basketball. My basketball friends and I were so focused on it, I paid very little attention to anything else.

The winter of my senior year, I continued with the same life-style. Football was over, and likely due to the concussions I received, the memory of the whole season is fleeting. Basketball season was here, and any form of partying would take a backseat. We fell one game short of making a run at state the previous year, and the team that beat us won it all. But thanks to our previous hard work, a great coach, and especially to my basketball friends, particularly one who would receive very high accolades, we went on to win the state title that year. I relished in the attention and praise that our small community gave for such an achievement. (I would love to carry on about this, but that is another story, and sharing it here could cause you to believe I peaked in high school.)

Spring of '88

Before my graduation, while everyone else was making plans for college or some type of continued education, I was … not. Indecision is a privilege of the young, but my time was drawing near. I believe I was too busy riding the high of our state title and still using this positive attention toward less constructive ideals. My coach informed me of a junior college that had offered somewhat of a scholarship for basketball, but I was reluctant. My thoughts of school were fleeting. Eventually, and in order to appease my parents and others, I said I would be attending a technical college for electric construction in the fall.

Summer arrived and I continued to party with what little money I had. And whatever I could convince my parents to give. I'm sure by now I must have been wearing my parents thin as the talk of finding a job seemed to be in every one of our conversations.

Luckily for them, a road construction company was working their way through town. My mother ran the local café in town at that time, and these construction workers had stopped and asked my mother if she knew anyone who needed a job. By noon that day, I was working road construction.

Fall of 1988

I enrolled myself into technical school. It was somewhat of a culture shock. I had no idea what to expect and had a hard time finding my place. I considered myself to be kind and sociable, but I was more comfortable around people who already knew me. My self-confidence was lacking. I hadn't really been anywhere yet, and the awkwardness was apparent and was beginning to cause me to search inward. I was missing the understanding of my friends and my free life. I stayed with my parents for a short time before making the move to the dorm rooms (apartments).

When I first moved in with a classmate from tech school, we attended keg parties and the like, but I never really felt a connection to anyone, including girls. Unbeknown to me at the time, I was truly beginning to feel the onset of what I now know to be depression—the internal negative dialogue. Having no girlfriend, no money, few friends, and time alone to reflect was not a good place for me.

CHAPTER 5

Complete Disclosure

(What happened in the short summer, school break of '89, will not soon be forgotten, if ever. Much contemplating was taken before I decided to involve this story. Surprisingly, the following experience has not risen to affect any part of my life since. I'm sure if I were to ever run for president, it would be very beneficial to my opponent. But in honor of the truth, I am choosing to leave it in.)

I was no stranger to the law at this age. Underage drinking had been on the rise currently, and I was one of many who acquired more than my share of arrests. I managed to create some type of ongoing conflict between myself and the local law enforcement but had yet to realize to what extent.

(What lies within the next few pages may be hard for you to fathom, just as hard as it is for me to openly explain. My credibility is likely at stake by this information. It is as personal as my depression and as equally difficult to explain. Please keep an open mind. I may just be overcompensating for years of holding back as nothing says "I no longer care what you think of me" like the blatant truth.)

I had issues with the law in my teenage years, but I was still unaware of the power they held. In the summer of 1989, I was again working road construction. One of my good friends and former teammate from high school and I decided to go to a street dance in a nearby town. For those who don't know, a street dance is just like it sounds. They block off the street so you can drink, dance, and watch a band play outside. It is most often done to celebrate a town's anniversary or to benefit a volunteer fire department or something of that nature. It is also a great environment for underage drinking to take place.

Toward the end of this evening, I witnessed a girl standing in the vicinity of my car. When I approached her, she looked to be a little younger than me but close in age. Our conversation led to her getting in the car with my friend and me. I made it abundantly clear as to where I lived and that I wouldn't be returning until the next day. Although it seemed odd to be so well trusted in such a short time; consider that I too, was still young and naïve.

She understood yet agreed to come with us. We dropped off my friend at his home and arrived at my parents' home. My room was in the basement of our ranch-style home, and my parents' room was indirectly above mine. Little did I know that the details of this evening, these specific details, would be gone over so discreetly and have such a potential dramatic impact on our future.

We did what you think we did, and I sensed nothing wrong when I awoke in the morning. I was listed as an alternate at a softball tournament, and it was possible that I would be asked to play the next day at her hometown. I called a friend to see if he wanted to accompany me for the day. The conversation between the three of us in the car seemed quite normal on the way back, but upon entering her hometown, she began to act apprehensive. She mentioned that her parents were probably looking for her, so she told me to drop her off about a block away from her home. I found this to be somewhat peculiar but truly didn't give it much thought at the time. The night before, she told me that she was nineteen and a half years old. She did say that she still lived with her parents and that they were extremely religious and very strict people.

I returned to my job with road construction on Monday morning. I was working about twenty miles from my parents' home. I believe it was the following Friday afternoon when a squad car pulled up. The officer asked me to stop at the courthouse after work. I agreed.

(Several months to a year prior, a friend of mine had some things stolen from him, and I had heard rumors and made speculations as to who may have done it. I had been in contact with the law, on the side of the law, off and on for several months regarding this issue, and I assumed this was the reason for our meeting.)

We sat down in his office as he began to ask a few questions. He seemed quite nervous and strange as he began asking if I knew a certain girl. I openly said I did, but then he said, "You are hereby charged with two counts of first-degree rape!" My stomach hit the floor. He proceeded to give me a short version of my Miranda rights and asked if I wanted to discuss this issue with him at this time. My distrust for the law and my prior courtroom experience told me that I obviously needed to see a lawyer before answering any more questions. A different officer appeared and placed handcuffs on me that were chained to a belt around my waist. He then led me outside to an awaiting patrol car.

My experience dealing with the law was not enough comfort to keep me from feeling the overwhelming anguish and anxiety about what was going to happen. My mind was racing back to the night in question, and all I could tell myself was that she must have lied about her age and was actually under sixteen. Not knowing the rules about rape or statutory rape at the time, I had no idea what to expect.

I was taken to the local detention center about thirty miles away. My only conversation with the officer driving was, "Look, man, I'm not a rapist. I don't belong in this car right now!"

His response, and quite possibly the only appropriate response, was, "If that is true, you will be released soon. Just have patience for the system."

We arrived at the detention center. Luckily, I looked like a typical hoodlum. I had an Ace wrap around my hand to cover the stitches I received from broken glass at work a few days prior. I was wearing camouflage pants and work boots. I was shirtless due to the heat and seemed to have forgotten to bring it amid the trauma of being arrested. I say I was lucky to look this way because I know it's best to fit in with your surroundings.

I was placed in medium security, where the alleged felons were held. I was obviously not comfortable there, but luckily, I was also a chameleon and had a way of blending in wherever I go. My paperwork was returned to me as I asked for my phone call. I tried desperately to contact my brother as I knew my parents were gone visiting relatives in Colorado. I needed a thousand dollars for bail, and I didn't have it. After many failed attempts, I contacted the waitress at my parents' café. Causing much panic and chaos, I eventually managed to get the message to my brother.

That night, I confided in my cell mate. We exchanged our stories and our mutual disgust for the law. (Of course, everyone in jail seems to have gotten a bum rap.) Seriously, he told me that it was probably best that I didn't tell anyone else the truth about my reasons for detention. He reminded me that some inmates might not believe in my innocence, and who knows why the rest were in here. Over breakfast, when asked "What are you in for," I told them I borrowed a car that was reported stolen (something I'd heard before).

The following morning, my brother arrived with the bail money. I was released, and on the way home, we discussed my situation. My brother assured me that there had been a mistake and that the 'idiots' in charge would eventually drop my case.

Finding peace at this moment was not an easy task. I believed I didn't break any laws, but judging my own history and the history of the law enforcement, anything could happen.

I would learn I was officially charged with two counts of first-degree rape, each carrying a maximum penalty of fifty years and fifty thousand dollars. I contacted a local law office in a neighboring county and explained the situation. My lawyer seemed young and inexperienced but had a convincing way of speaking. I'm sure I was his biggest case at that time. He seemed to work more on the side of sympathy and truth rather than the cold, calculated, and heartless way of some lawyers you might imagine. After meeting face-to-face and hearing my story, he looked me in the eye and said, "You're not guilty."

I immediately fired back "Ya think? This is my life hanging in the balance, and I can't have someone defending me who doesn't believe me!"

"I believe you," he assured.

My lawyer informed me of the current rules regarding rape in our state. Statutory rape, at this time, was when an adult had sex with a minor fifteen years of age or younger. First-degree rape was forced sex or sex without the partner's ability to give consent due to mental incapacity. Since her age was actually sixteen, they pursued first-degree rape. They based their case on the argument that she was not capable of giving consent to sex due to intoxication. 'Date rape' is what it is referred to now but this lesser sanction didn't exist at the time. My defense would now be based on whether or not she was sober enough to give consent. It would be months before my actual trial.

I was now on a roller coaster of emotions. I felt confident after meetings with my lawyer and witnesses, but during the alone time, my vivid and dangerous imagination began to contemplate prison and what happened to rapists, guilty or not.

Tech school became somewhat of hobby now as I was rarely attending. I would spend a week or two in a depressive state until I would eventually give in socially to friends and carry on. And now that I, myself am currently a parent, I cannot fathom the stress I induced upon my parents.

The Trial

I was up against my newest and worst enemies: the justice system. I had somehow, in the course of my younger days, starting with my minibike, developed certain hatred between myself and the local law enforcement, a hatred that would reveal itself during the beginning stages of my trial. The sheriff who arrested me was on the stand and changing his stories and fabricating his own right in front of our eyes. My outraged friend and witness immediately pointed out an obvious lie to my lawyer and during the cross-examination, the sheriff on the stand began to show physical signs of his dishonesty. Like a little kid guilty of stealing cookies, he began to rub the arm of the chair while his eyes wandered about. It was obvious to all who witnessed that he had just perjured himself. It was a positive attribute to my case yet left me with an uneasy feeling. I couldn't believe the extent they were willing to go to see me put away. What kind of person did they think I was? They were truly willing to lie and see me put away before admitting a mistake.

The incompetence on the state's side would soon reveal itself. The state's attorney, at one point, cross-examined my character witness, asking her if she was there the night in question. She replied in a calm voice, "No, I'm a character witness." My lawyer objected eventually and explained to the judge that she was here to give witness to my character and not the night in question. The way I understand, there is usually no need or desire to cross-examine a character witness. The judge agreed and shook his head in disgust. The ineptitude was obvious.

The next couple days of the trial were the most difficult. Having to give detail to a sexual encounter in front of strangers, let alone your parents, is an extremely difficult task. I can vividly remember the look on some of the elderly ladies' faces in the jury. I could see and hear their displeasure when certain words were mentioned. My lawyer reassured me as he explained that just sex out of wedlock seemed foreign to some of the older jury members.

Coming from or going to recess, I remember making eye contact with the alleged victim. Without drawing attention to myself, I mouthed the word *why*. She looked away just as quickly.

Eventually, it seemed that everyone involved had taken the stand, including a couple friends of the alleged victim. They stated through allowed hearsay that they had heard the alleged victim state that she was intentionally going out that night to 'get back at her parents'.

My lawyer reassured the jury that forced sex did not happen and was not in question even though the opposition liked to bring it up. Having the ability to give consent was in question, and when the alleged victim took the stand, she was asked how much alcohol she had consumed. Thankfully, she seemed to give a fairly honest testimony.

My lawyer and I summoned an alcohol specialist to give an educated depiction as to her level of sobriety. Accounting for her body weight and amount of alcohol consumed, he found her to be approximately close to the illegal amount for driving while having sex that evening. But in the morning, during intercourse the second time, it was proven that she had almost no alcohol in her system. It deemed a huge attribute to my case.

It was left in the hands of the jury. I had visions of the worst. I was afraid for myself and for my parents and what they were going through. I was standing outside the courthouse for about ten minutes when my lawyer retrieved me. He had a positive look on his face as he felt that the less time a jury would spend in deliberation, the better our chances.

"Please rise."

I stood to hear the verdict. I was inert. I could feel the weakness in my legs. Sounds began to echo in my head. I developed tunnel vision as I questioned my consciousness. I kept my hand on the chair in front me. I had to remind myself to breath.

In my twisted mind, I briefly contemplated the height of the third-floor window of the courtroom. I envision jumping headfirst and question if it would be enough to end me. I quickly thought about the physical stunts that I'd undertaken in the past and realized that it wouldn't be near enough. These brief suicidal thoughts were interrupted by the jury foreman. He stood and read aloud, "We, the jury, find the defendant not guilty".

I could hear my mother gasp behind me. I hugged her tightly and said, "It's over, Mom! It's okay." My next hug was for my lawyer.

A few days later, I would hear rumors that the alleged victim's family asked to drop the case halfway through the trial. The state's attorney obviously recommended against it. The family was told that I could sue for defamation of character if it didn't continue to the end—his only good advice. My trial and lawyer costs came to the tune of about ten thousand dollars, a personal loan from the bank. I asked my lawyer if there was any way I could sue the state for this amount. He informed me that it was possible but could end up costing more than that amount to win.

Looking back, I can understand her parents' misdirected anger. I can understand the fear and trepidation that had to inhabit the girl's mind, being raised in such a strict environment. I blame the only people deserving, the state's attorney and law enforcement, for pursuing this case and convincing her family to pursue it as well.

Did I do something morally wrong? Definitely. Did I break the law? Hell no!

(According to my math, if I were to have been found guilty and sentenced, I would likely just be getting out, if I survived. And the law wonders why I sometimes take the side of the alleged criminal.)

Surprisingly, having had such a tragic event, I have yet to realize that lifestyle forecasts consequence. How easy it is to distract one's self from problems by the unconscious creation of more.

CHAPTER 6

Friends

So much for sitting down and pounding this out. This is not the pace. Some of this was written years ago. Other than one Advil pm, I am still sober. The Patriots play Denver today for AFC championship. I don't have an opinion. I had a glimpse of Depression a few days ago, other than that, doing well. Temps are in high 70s here and 20s back home with an occasional snowstorm. Have to go back in about 80 days. Get to work.

—January 19, 2014, daily
journal (unedited)

My moment

There comes a moment within the day, when I
    don't think before I say,
But the eye of my mind begins to wander.
In search of reason so discrete, in search of doubt
    that is concrete,
To bury this moment under.
This confusion takes anchor in ways of frustration
In order to steal what has already passed.
And I take this with me, the unfounded awareness,
That this moment would never last.

INSIGHT

> The question that's always hazy,
> am I or the others crazy?

> —Einstein

In the fall of '89, I returned to school. Kale was again off working various jobs—building grain bins, helping farmers, and at one point, working with his father for a construction/excavating company. Kale invited the challenge of physical labor and took pride in proving himself. He never had a problem finding work. I would still see him on occasion, and when I did, we would continue to party like rock stars, if allowed. Kale would return from wherever he was, and we would start our day off by picking up a twelve-pack and driving around on the gravel roads. Sometimes we would fish or hunt, but I was mostly there for conversation and his stories from the road. Pot entered the equation from time to time, and the humor that ensued may be beyond my ability to express.

I'd never been a stranger to marijuana, yet I rarely went out of my way to obtain it. My greaser friends considered me to be a mooch (I rarely had my own). If it showed itself and conditions were right, I had no problem with it. I looked at it as an enhancer. For me, it seemed to accentuate whatever emotions I was having. Although I indulged in everything, I believe in the theory "All things in moderation." Right?

Kale's sense of humor matched well with mine and seemed to work on a level most bystanders could not understand. We shared a very deep mind-set, and knowing each other so well, much of the humor instigated was understood without verbalizing. During interactions with others, his approach was more the way of sly innuendos, while mine was more friendly and unassuming. If we happened to be high in a small crowd of people, our silly, uncontrollable laughter often left others unable to 'get it', and judging by the looks on their faces, we also left them with the belief that we were not from this planet. Inconspicuous comedy came easy to us. I also seemed to lose all inhibition in his presence. His confidence was contagious.

Kale had a way of discovering the addressee's personal disturbing and internalized emotions during conversation. He slowly, mischievously exploited these sentiments until the recipient of this emotional bullying would eventually notice our deception, to which they would abruptly pause midsentence and defensively reply "Fuck you!" Just as quickly, Kale would respond, usually leaning in with a hand on the shoulder and chuckling, "Sorry, man! Just givin' ya shit!" It almost always ended in laughter from both parties. Kale understood empathy; he just used it as a means to provoke and later make light of the issue to possibly get them to witness their own behavior and acknowledge their own absurd thoughts; to get them to be their true selves. In Kale's presence, it was not only recommended that you be yourself—it was required. I doubt he knew what he was doing at the time, but in a roundabout way, in my eyes, he was saying, "You think *you've* got problems?"

In time, I have learned that this provocative behavior, although rare, does in fact seem to loosen and open people up at a much faster rate than if one had to be cordial—as a means to unburden them. Be real. Be honest. No substitute behavior allowed. Those who were possibly too sensitive and never did see the humor had the tendency to walk away. Those who recognized their own absurdity seemed to feel liberated, at least temporarily. I know I always did when it was applied to me.

I had always thought I lacked the ability to express myself accurately, and Kale seemed the exact opposite—often socially inappropriate but always brutally honest. Even during sobriety, he often took things to an extreme measure. But with the aid of alcohol or pot, to me he was reality's comedian. Rarely embarrassed, straightforward, and at times confrontational, he always, without fear, seemed to create many uncomfortable challenges for those around him. He had a tendency to quickly bring out the best or the worst in people. These episodes would happen anywhere and everywhere we went, but our favorite place to be was Rob's.

Closed many years ago, there was a bar in a neighboring town where the owner still believed the drinking age should be eighteen. "Old enough to die for your country, you're old enough to drink in my bar," he'd say under his breath. The owner, Rob, was an unsightly fellow. Some stories say that he was born with dwarfism, but it was also believed that he had broken his back falling down the stairs at a young age. It just seemed too personal to ask him. He resembled a hunchback. He wore a black beard and spoke like the famous old disc jockey Wolf man Jack. Oddly, he also reminded me of Angus Young, the lead singer of ACDC.

I make no apologies for the way I speak of him as brutal honestly was also his language. He stood around maybe five feet tall, was fairly humble and quiet, yet had a forceful, abrasive way of speaking that commanded respect. Strangers rarely labeled him a nice guy, yet almost everyone who frequented his bar loved him like a brother. He loved truth and seemed to think compliments and politeness were a waste of time. If you did catch him alone, he would eventually reveal his softer side.

Kale seemed to really enjoy conversations with Rob. He also looked up to some of the townspeople. Everyone here seemed to have a nickname with a story behind all of them. They too considered themselves to be greasers, more of an adult version. I was younger than most, and they all seemed to know my parents, whom they considered to be more 'normal', for the lack of a better word. At first, they seemed reluctant to express themselves in front of me while in their presence. It was Kale's bold informalities that bridged the gap, and he did this often, likely without intention. The locals also knew that the entertainment value in their favorite bar always increased with Kale's presence.

Kale and I would always end up at Rob's no matter where we started our day. Besides it being the only bar I could drink in at the time, I would find the confrontations and jovial hostilities between all of us to be hilarious. We would catch a buzz outside and come inside to play video games and eat munchies from the bar. Rob would follow us around and bitch while he cleaned up our messes of cheese popcorn and Reese's. He'd watch us laugh hysterically playing the football game where you had to frantically and continuously punch down a button as fast as you could to make your player run. In the heat of the game, while running for a touchdown, we'd usually knock one another off the barstools in order to cheat. Rob would shake his head in disgust. "Fuckin' kids!" he'd mumble. Even if Kale wasn't with me, I would often find myself at this bar to get my monthly dose of truth from Rob and the locals.

In tech school, I met and quickly became friends with an African American who called himself Cee. We played basketball together for our school, and we seemed to enjoy one another's company. A few selected friends would eventually coin us as 'salt and pepper', most likely due to the fact we were living in what Cee referred to as a 'white man's world'. Cee and I seemed to take the nickname in stride. We did have a lot in common. We both liked break dancing, basketball, and smoking weed occasionally. I looked forward to introducing my new friend to my best friend.

Kale called on a Thursday. He informed me that he'd recently bought a new car (new to him) and wanted to go for a road trip. I told him to pick me and my new friend up at my apartment. I was patiently waiting when I heard a motor revving outside at an extreme rate, enough to 'float the valves'. I looked outside, and Kale was sitting in a 1970(?) Dodge Satellite, stomping on the accelerator. I had explained our evening plans with Cee earlier, and as I pointed out the window, I said, "Well, there's our ride!" Prior to this, I had given a brief description of my friend as a 'dirty white boy', and the concerned look Cee gave me as he looked out the window would quickly confirm my description.

Upon entering the vehicle, Kale exclaimed, "Buckle up, boys, this thing's got balls!" Lacking better judgment, we reluctantly sat down. I asked him if was drunk. He quickly replied, "Not yet!"

We pulled out onto the highway, and within a half mile, before reaching sixty miles per hour, we were out of control. He had somehow hooked the shoulder of the road and slid into a fortunately, smooth and manageable ditch. Slowing to a stop and bumping into a fence post, he immediately looked over and said, "Shit, Johnny, maybe you better drive!" We looked in the backseat at Cee. With arms stretched from door to door, he instantly agreed.

We made our way to Rob's. Through booze and the occasional toke on a pipe, we all got along well. Closing time came and on our way back to my place (me driving), a racial discussion took place between Kale and Cee. Cee mentioned that during the course of the night, through a conversation with one of the locals, he felt the guy was being racist. Knowing the local and having heard some of their conversation, Kale quickly became upset. He said, "You can't make a blanket statement like that if you don't know him! Just because you sensed that the guy didn't agree with you or like you doesn't make him a racist. Judging someone because they don't believe what you believe or don't agree with you makes *you* prejudice! I have the freedom to choose who I like, black, white, or whatever, and if I don't like you, it's probably because you're just an asshole!" Pausing and now pointing his finger at Cee, he continued, "And don't think for a minute that because of the color of your skin, you get to judge anyone!"

Cee was definitely not a small, timid man, but he didn't seem to argue long over this subject tonight as he could tell how making hasty judgments of others seemed to infuriate Kale. When they parted ways, they shook hands and shared a quick 'bro hug'. Within a few days, Cee was asking, "When do we get to see the dirty white boy again?"

That's the irony of Kale—prone to violent outbursts when he considered himself in the right, yet doesn't want anyone acting judgmental. He loved to be the underdog and fight for the underdog; the strong arm of moral law violently working toward peace.

Within the following months, I would find my grades to be irreparable due to many absences during my prior trial and my mental detachment. I would eventually drop out before making the extra effort to graduate. I made plans to retake a few classes again the following year. My recently developed desire for money would cause me to return to my road construction job. The average electrician pay was about six dollars per hour at this time. Road construction paid around ten dollars to fifteen dollars per hour, depending on what machine you operated. Overtime pay was also likely.

In the summer of 1990, now again working road construction and currently living with my sister and her family a short distance from home, working twelve hour days and most weekends left little time for play. I had met a girl through a friend and we'd become quite close; my first real relationship since high school. Her parents lived close by, but she was attending college about eight hours away. Through her patience and extreme tolerance, we managed to stay together for almost a year. My selfishness and alcohol abuse caused many complications in our relationship. I seemed to drop everything I was doing, including her, whenever the opportunity to party with Kale or anyone else came about. Kale would return from the road on occasion and when it was possible, we'd continue barhopping along with our gravel-road stories. My childish ways and constant desire to be entertained seemed to supersede everything else. It was obvious that I was far too immature to maintain a serious relationship. After a few relationship mistakes, her parents wisely threatened to stop paying for her college education if she continued to see me. She would make the right choice.

But I felt it. It was the first time in my life as an adult, and since puppy love, that a matter of the heart, something this conflicting and severe, could not be worked out in my favor. I acknowledged this fact shortly after and briefly began to question my own behavior for the first time. This too was short-lived, however, as I was only twenty now, and showing concern for my future was still not part of my plan because I had no plan. To me, becoming self-aware without having a plan is not truly self-awareness.

Luckily, the few friends I did make while attending tech school had witnessed me working road construction locally and asked if I wanted to try electrical work. They worked nearby, and although I would be taking a serious pay cut, I reluctantly took the job.

Now working forty hours a week, having weekends free, made ample time for the things I truly enjoyed. Kale had purchased his own home back in our hometown. I was almost twenty-one, my rent was cheap, and I often returned home to raid my parents' fridge and party with Kale.

It was a typical Saturday. We'd start about noon. Kale pulled into my parents' driveway in a '70s pacer. You know, the car that resembled a bubble and was prone to blow up in flames when bumped from the rear. It was obviously missing a muffler. Smiling, he stepped out of one of the ugliest cars known to man and boldly asked, "Guess what I paid for it?"

"Whatever it was, you got took!" I replied.

"Come on, man!" He offered, "This thing's got a jeep chassis!"

I sat down in the passenger seat. Luckily, I was wearing work clothes. The car was filthy inside and out. "Sorry 'bout the mess. Been using it as a work car!" he announced with laughter.

There was an open twelve-pack in the backseat. Discarded mail and cans littered the floor.

"I got this bitch for a hundred bucks!" he exclaimed. "You believe that?"

"Well, yeah, it's a piece o' shit!" I replied.

"Hey! Wait 'til you ride in her before you start bad-mouthin' her!"

"Where we goin'?" I asked.

"Who cares?" He shrugged. "I got a full tank of gas and money in my pocket!"

Who could resist?

I don't recall the order in which he would arrive in one of his many 'paycheck' cars (a car that is fully paid for by less than a one-week paycheck). It happened frequently, and he was always just as enthused about each one. This type of temporary car was very suitable for those of us who work construction, and Kale relished in the fact that he could run through and over obstacles on the road and not worry about scratching his paint. He also explained that if his coffee got cold on the way to work, he could just dump it on the passenger floor so he wouldn't have to open a window. If your ashtray was full, you could stuff out your smoke in the same place—unconventional but appropriate. He enjoyed a certain unique freedom driving such expendable vehicles, and concern for his appearance never seemed to be an issue. I believe he understood the disconcerted looks he would get when he'd pull up in such a vehicle, as if he dared you to make a comment. (Kale was the guy you'd see at the gas station who pulled up with a loud, obnoxious piece of shit car, and as you were about to form a disgusted look on your face, he stepped out to look right at you while you quickly revert to giving him a passive smile and nod of approval.)

We drive away in this 'bubble' car and encountered my current insurance agent on the street, an acquaintance of ours from the same school. He pompously walked up to Kale's window, and with a nervous tone, knowing he might be risking it, he sarcastically commented, "Nice car, Kale."

Sensing the sarcasm, pointing down at his shoes, Kale instantly replied, "You're just jealous 'cause you paid more for your sneakers than I paid for a whole car!" As our acquaintance looked down at his pearly-white tennis shoes, he quickly tried to lighten the mood and explain his comment. But before he could muster a word, Kale revved the exhaustless motor and pulled away. Looking back in the mirror and laughing, he left him standing in a cloud of smoke.

It was not rare to see this amount of confidence and pride within obvious self-deprecating humor. It seems to state "I know who I am, and I will not be deterred by your opinion of me." He was very proud of his greaser status. Yeah, Kale was cocky, but it seemed more of a justified self-confidence. He was an intelligent, good-looking and misunderstood badass. This was a time in his life when he saw himself as who he was, and made us aware of it.

I arrive at a bar. The place was rather full as some people had spilled out onto the sidewalk. I approached Kale. Our conversation led to our mutual friend, Dave.

"Where *is* Dave?" I inquired.

He pointed to the bar, "I think he's inside. I'm kinda surprised they haven't kicked him out yet."

"Why's that? Is he drunk?"

Giggling, he replied, "Yeah, pretty fucked up—obnoxious!"

Just then, as if on cue, the door to the bar swung open, and out came Dave with a guy on top of him, clinging to him. The man had Dave by the hair now as Dave ended up on the sidewalk on all fours. He punched Dave on the back of the head while cursing. Dave replied, "Go ahead and hit me on the back of the head! You can't hurt me!"

My eyes quickly focused on Kale to see his reaction. He was attentive but hesitant to help. He and Dave were close, but we both knew that our close friend often deserved a couple of knots on the head. Dave ultimately scrambled to his feet. He lunged at the guy, but the guy eluded him. The next scene, my larger friend, Dave, was now chasing this smaller man down the street until the amused crowd finally lost interest.

A few minutes later, my attention was brought again toward Kale. He was currently in a heavy discussion with friends of the man Dave was fighting. They were standing between two cars parked about six feet apart. Missing the beginning of the conversation, I heard the man say, "You're not fast enough!" With that, Kale sent out two fast right-hand jabs that stopped within a half inch of the man's nose.

"That ain't fast enough?" Kale replied. Within seconds, the man lurched forward, with both hands grabbing Kale's jacket toward his neck. Kale released a flurry of short combinations including inside hooks and uppercuts until the man fell back on the hood of the car. Two men standing adjacent to Kale instantly grabbed Kale's arms to hold him back while the man quickly regained himself to an upright position. For a second, I felt the sensation that happens when you think you're going to have to intervene. It would appear Kale was now in trouble. The man gathered himself to lurch forward at Kale again. While still in the grasp, Kale sent a snapping front kick that connected with his face. The witnesses all let out a collective moan as the man fell back on the car. As if in shock by the instant brutality, the two guys loosened their grip. Kale shook himself loose and repositioned to the sidewalk in a fighting stance directed toward the two who intervened. Blood was already running down the hood of the car and onto the front bumper. Kale's brother Steve was in attendance and immediately told Kale to leave before the cops arrived. Kale relaxed from his stance, took a slow look around, reached down and grabbed his beer that he somehow remembered was sitting on the bumper, and then quickly disappeared around the corner.

The following weekend, Kale was working on his recently purchased Harley-Davidson. It was a late-seventies sportster, and we were all secretly glad that it had mechanical problems. In a condescending tone, I mentioned to Kale that I heard the guy he thumped required almost a hundred stitches. Intentionally dodging my point, he looked up from his work at his fists. Carefully examining them, he replied, "I know. It's like I have razor blades for knuckles!" After we share a quick laugh, he acknowledged my inquisition as he knew why I mentioned it. He then stared at me to say "Hey ... he had a chance to walk away. He knew he was gonna fight when he tried to grab me. Tough shit if he didn't know what he was in for!"

It was a typical Friday night. I arrived at Rob's expecting to see Kale. He was not around. I asked Rob if he'd seen him. He informed me that he was here and left. He went on to tell me that a few of our friends, Kale's and mine, were in Rob's earlier and received a phone call from a bar they were just in, where they were accused of stealing someone's darts. Kale, having not been with them but equally offended by the accusations, offered to ride along while they went back to confront the accusers.

I sat and drank with Rob. After a couple of hours, they returned. Walking in with enthusiastic smiles on their faces, the men from the group sat down and began to share details of the melee that took place and inform Rob of their individual fights. I listened intently. One of the girls from the group, a classmate of Kale's from high school, sat next to me with this astonished look. I knew her well, and I asked her what happened. Taking a deep breath, she replied, "That was the craziest shit I've ever seen! There were three fights happening all at the same time!" Pointing at Kale, she stated, "He basically kicked the shit out of two guys!" I told her to calm down and fill me in.

She informed me of the accusations and the reasons they returned to the bar. She said, "When we got there, before we even got out of the vehicle, Kale pointed his finger to the guys in the backseat and said, 'We ain't goin in there to talk! Get it in your fuckin heads right now that you're in a fight!'" She went on, "When we walked in, Kale grabbed a guy and the shit was on! Jimmy had a guy! Merle had a guy! And even Merle's sister was in on it, fighting one their girlfriends! Although she kinda got her ass kicked." She struggled with the details but at the end of our talk, lowering her voice as she nodded toward Kale, she proclaimed, "That is one tough son of a bitch!"

When I finally spoke with Kale, he told me that he had to pay attention to more than one guy at a time and that the details were sketchy. Under his breath, he also mentioned that he may have even thrown a girl who tried to stop it into the wall at one point. Instead of trying to recall particulars, he seemed more proud of the fact that when it was basically over, some guy threw a metal napkin holder at him. Reenacting the move, he said, "I swatted it right outta the air like fuckin Bruce Lee!"

Hours later at Rob's, when all was calm, intermittently still discussing the night's events, Kale was now fairly drunk. He looked at me intently as he quietly stated under his breath so no one else could hear, "I know you think fightin' is wrong, Johnny, and you don't like to see people get fucked up. And that's good. But I have to tell you, right or wrong, I'm pretty damn good at it!"

Kale was a self-proclaimed fallen angel. It was literally written on his arm. He seemed beyond reproach. Most often, there was a logical excuse or reason for his actions. When there was no excuse or reason, he was quick to defend ideals, and it was easily understood that this was just who he was.

I often believe badasses can spot other badasses quickly, and therefore, tend to know who's capable and who's not. So they seem to lose fights less often, possibly the act of understanding the hierarchy of the herd. Or maybe it's their straightforward, confident approach to conversations. People avoid confrontations with them because they instantly know where they stand. But this isn't the movies. If you fight often, you will eventually lose. Kale would admit to taking a beating on occasion and would give credit where credit was due. He would make the obvious excuses as to being too drunk or outnumbered at times and he was also quick to admit if he had a beating coming.

Kale's brother Daniel told him years ago that if you do get your ass kicked, the next day, you have to ask yourself this question—can I live it down? He meant that you had to objectively look at the situation. Did you provoke it? Did the guy honorably defend himself? Or was he the instigator? Was it fair? Were you both ready? Answer these questions before you decide to retaliate. Can you walk away from it in your mind? Look at it for what it is without anger, and see if you can you live it down. This is thoughtful advice on how to move on.

When I once asked Kale for advice on how to not get your ass kicked, he stated, "The first thing helpful to know about winning a fight is to be the first to know you're in one." Kale usually had to get shoved or swung at before unloading. But his experience taught him to never assume it was going to end peacefully. Your odds are always better when you're not playing defense.

Street fights seemed to be an understood lifestyle for many in this era. Luckily, this was a time before cell phones or before many people carried weapons. It was also a time where it seemed dishonorable to throw cheap shots. I'm sure they happened, but it seemed to be an unwritten code among a majority of local bar fighters that you first called someone outside, like in an old West movie. Kale said pussies would throw cheap shots, and unless you were facing unreasonable odds, you rarely would send a blindside punch. I agree. And there's really no law broken when two people agree to settle an argument with violence, at least not morally. But not everyone follows unwritten rules. And to live this way is extremely dangerous. It was surprising how many wanted to confront Kale even though they'd heard similar stories. There seemed to be many who attempted to dethrone him. Some people seek attention no matter what form it may be.

I have never condemned nor condoned Kale for his violent streaks. We would often discuss the fights later, and as much as he would conceal it, I could tell he was remorseful. What amazed me about the prior incident (the guy who required many stitches) was the fact that Kale remembered where his beer was immediately after the fight. Among the chaos and the emotional and physical drama of such a barbaric confrontation, he calmly remembered and relocated a half-empty can of beer. It had now become clear to me that in Kale's mind, violence seemed as natural as kindness.

By now, I'm sure you've been asking yourself just what is it that draws me to such a person—prone to violence, overbearing, and sometimes, just plain rude. How is it that I chose Kale's company over others? I'm sure my friends often asked themselves the same question. Kale was not a man of many words, just the right ones. Our conversations usually consisted of me doing most of the talking, asking philosophical questions. At this time in my life, I was still searching for this thing that propelled others. I am determined to solve the riddle: "what makes us who we are?". I was still trying to emulate self-confidence, self-assurance, and a lifestyle that I felt I was in charge of. Amid the drunken chaos and disarray, I might have been slowly, unconsciously discovering myself. And maybe others' problems were also a distraction to my own as I had yet to take responsibility for myself.

Whether Kale was right or wrong, I was drawn to his conviction. I had always struggled with confrontation and making impulse decisions. I tended to regret more of what I did not do than what I'd done. I admit that I was also fascinated by physical confrontation because of the truth that lay within; that however barbaric and brutal it could be to inflict pain upon another, the decision to be physically violent was the finality of the disagreement- the true end of conversation. Enough said.

Kale and I would debate often over the issues of peace and violence. Kale's violent tendencies likely originated during childhood. If you grew up having to fight for survival, you would unavoidably use violence often. Neither of us had ever directed this behavior toward women or children or those incapable of defending themselves. Both of us were raised better than that. Yet becoming this product of your environment is very difficult to deny. Kale claimed that violence ruled the world. I argued that intelligence rules the world.

We were driving through main street in our local college town in my rusted out Chevy Blazer one afternoon while debating this same topic. I saw two men briskly walking the sidewalk, wearing suits, and each carrying a briefcase (likely lawyers leaving their office—we were in that vicinity). My current claim was that the rich and educated would rule the world. Pointing at the two suits, I exclaimed to Kale, "Those guys rule the world."

In Kale's instant response, he replied, "No they don't. Watch this." While rolling down his window, he stuck his head outside, put on his mean face and aggressive tone, and shouted, "Hey!" Just as soon as the two stopped to turn their heads in our direction, Kale continued, "What-are-you lookin-at?!" Just as quickly, they fearfully turned back around and continued walking, wanting nothing to do with us. Laughing, Kale turned back to me. "Ha-ha! See? Violence still rules the world." I would lose this round.

CHAPTER 7

Be Here Now

The only people for me are the mad ones, the ones who are mad to live, mad to talk, mad to be saved, desirous of everything at the same time, the ones who never yawn or say a commonplace thing, but burn, burn, burn like fabulous yellow roman candles exploding like spiders across the stars."

—Jack Kerouac, *On the Road*

During the last couple of years and since Kale's move back to our hometown, his reputation had now truly been established. The company he kept seemed to instigate trouble and violence on occasion. He was obviously never a stranger to violence and was known for having a quick trigger figuratively and literally. It was not something you would mistake if you met him as it was clearly recognizable in his aura. But acquaintances often feared being around him for several reasons: He could be defensive at times, and just knowing his past violent encounters, they would safely direct their attention elsewhere. He also had the tendency to 'ruffle your feathers' during conversation by belittling your problems. Kale's closer friends and I could handle the disparagement as we knew he would never physically harm us, even though we knew he was very capable. He and I sparred and wrestled enough to make that perfectly clear. I saw enough of him to know that out of all the fights he was in, the majority did take place while in defense of a friend. I'm sure he likely caused some due to boredom, alcohol, or in essence, claiming your territory. It was a normal thing back then to be involved in some type of skirmish on many weekends. Kale rarely sought trouble while in my presence, but carrying yourself in such an audacious way has a tendency to offend many strangers, and if you dared to instigate a physical confrontation, he would likely oblige.

I had no problem pissing Kale off. When he would randomly tell me a story and mispronounce or use the wrong words entirely and being the English stickler that I claimed to be, I'd reprimand him. He'd pause to look at me and say, "Hey, did you know what I meant? Yeah? Then shut the fuck up!" (The point is the point).

Kale would also tire of hearing me receiving praises from the locals in bars about our recent state championship in basketball. He had to find out for himself if I was as good as people thought I was. Whenever he'd mention kickin' my ass, I'd respond with, "Well, you're a fighter. I'm a basketball player. Try me at what I do best." We set the drinking aside one afternoon and found the nearest outside court. We continued until we were both exhausted. We lost track of the score and fouls as I ended up with a bloody nose. If it wasn't for my outside shooting, he may have even beaten me. Kale didn't do anything half-assed. I accepted his only compliment while we drove away. "Not bad, not bad, Johnny!" The beer tasted a little better that night.

Kale and I challenged each other often with contests to establish our manhood. We stopped in front his mother's driveway one evening while we were both tuned up and feeling cocky. I was usually hesitant to spar with him, as even taking an accidental hit from Kale was painful. We'd wrestled many times, but it had been a while since we sparred. Tonight I was more aggressive, and we ended up throwing hard body punches. After taking a few shots, when he was within range, on instinct and likely out of fear, I gave him a quick combination to his forehead. He immediately subdued me onto the ground. I hollered, "I'm done! I'm done!" Thankfully, he was likely shocked by this retaliation and didn't continue to pummel me. He was likely just trying to see what I was capable of as we did this a few times. While we reentered the car, Kale checked himself out in the rear-view mirror. Chuckling, he announced, "Christ! It's like I got hit by a jackhammer!" A couple knots later appeared on his forehead and when questioned by our friends at the local bar, he proudly said, "Yeah, don't fuck with Johnny!"

He was a harmless bully to his friends. The type of guy to knock your hat off, and when you bend over to pick it up, laughing, he would push you. When you'd get mad and make a fist, he'd oblige by turning his shoulder toward you. Flexing, he offered a target. When you put a cigarette in your mouth, before you could light it, he'd slap it out and send it flying. He bored easily. There were times when these acts would offend you, but there was no denying the humor. I often returned these actions in the same way every chance I could just because it was simply that damn funny. Kale also didn't seem to mind this behavior when he found himself on the receiving end.

Amid Kale's often domineering behavior, there were underlying complexities to him and I was gradually becoming the person with whom he would confide. We were beginning to argue more frequently as I seemed to be exempted from any serious physical confrontation. And our protégé-mentor relationship was now becoming more equal. I was no longer intimidated by him mentally. During our 3:00 a.m. gravel-road conversations, he was beginning to show signs of inner turmoil. I had seen indications of this previously but was slowly becoming more aware of it. He was asking me to listen more intently now as he was beginning to respect my advice as I had always respected his. He was still currently heartbroken over his ex-girlfriend and their son. He often missed his brother Daniel. He wondered why the rest of his family didn't seem to want him to love his father. (We would regretfully remind him of how his father once treated him.) We talked about God, life and death, and women and their complications. He was truly sincere at these times, and before he would tell a story, he would regularly ask, "Are you my friend?" I was usually a very good listener. When I dropped him off after a night of these deep conversations, he often shook my hand while looking straight into my eyes as he stated, "You're my best friend, Johnny!"

If we were out partying together, assuming I was too drunk or just way too distracted to listen, or if our moods were not cohesive, he would tell me, "Hey! Be here now!" (I would find out much later that this phrase was taken from a book he'd recently read with that said title by Ram Dass, *Be Here Now*.) With that ferocious stare, pointing his finger in my face, he would explain it in his own way. "Hey! Whoever you are, Johnny, I need you to *be* you right fucking *here* and right fucking *now*!" This phrase came in handy to get someone's undivided attention. He would usually follow it up with a heartfelt story. Many of these stories seemed to center around his complications with his ex-girlfriend and his son, mostly in the direction of how he wished they could be together as a family.

While out on these gravel roads at 3:00 a.m., after a heavy discussion on the rights and wrongs of love and hate in this world, he would attempt feats so as to distract his mind. He would suddenly stop the car on a bridge overlooking a frozen creek about ten feet down.

It was the middle of winter, and the temperature was well below zero with the wind chill. It was already tempting fate to be out here in these elements. This bridge's railings angled toward the top about twelve to fifteen feet above the road. He proceeded to climb up and swing out using just his hands. In front of the headlights, I watched him as he moved hand over hand the thirty-foot distance of the bridge and dropped back onto the road. When he got back into the car, I asked, "What the hell was that about?"

As he shook the cold from his hands, he replied, "Whoa! I just had to get a different state of mind ... Gimme a beer!"

When Kale's coworkers were home from the road, his similar feats often preceded him. I once heard someone bet Kale a hundred dollars he couldn't climb the underside of the stairway that encompassed a forty-foot grain bin. They placed a rock on top of a hundred-dollar bill and left it at the top step. Using just his hands, on the backside of jagged steps of the stairway, he climbed hand over hand. He not only impressed the onlookers by climbing it, but while at the top, he also grabbed the hundred, stuffed it in his pocket, tossed the rock, and climbed down the same way. Later, when I brought this to

Kale's attention, I questioned those actions. He told me that he didn't have the energy to get around the steps, so he had to climb down the same way. This physical feat would require several stitches on his hands. I then asked how much it cost for the stitches. Laughing, he replied, "About a hundred bucks!"

I would inquire about these physical feats and risky behavior as there were more than I can mention. Kale told me that he always felt better afterward. He said that the adrenaline rush and the physical exertion seemed to be the quickest way to 'get right'. There was much truth to his theory, although jogging proves to be much safer.

21

My twenty-first birthday found me living in our college town. I was currently working as an apprentice electrician for a local contractor here. I call it a college town due to the extreme transformation during summers. The population dropped in half when school let out. In the summer, it would near twenty thousand but would basically double during the school year. My brother also lived in this town at the time and worked at a local factory. For extra cash on the weekends, we also painted barns, outbuildings, and houses inside and out.

Kale was back from the road for a holiday and I invited him to "grace land," my current home, for a house party. I was somewhat apprehensive about the evening. I was expecting somewhat of a clash between the so-shez and the greasers. My college friends all came from similar small towns but were not considered wealthy. Many of them had taken out school loans and were trying to find the balance between studying and partying. They referred to me as a 'townie'. Although Kale could be somewhat abrasive and often way too direct, he'd always been very respectful of my parents and my close friends. He seemed to be on his best behavior if I reminded him. "Don't raise hell with 'em. I have to live here," I'd tell him. I informed my roommates that a friend of mine was on his way over and to keep an eye out for him because he'd never been here before.

Several of us were standing outside in our front yard drinking keg beer. It was dark out, yet our streets were pretty well lit. We noticed a beat-up blue Chevette pull up across the street. It was Kale (never knew what he was going to be driving). We took notice because he just pulled onto the curb and back down again so as to avoid parallel parking. He seemed unaware of our presence as he had never been to grace land. He opened the door and set his personal beer on the hood and the rest of his twelve-pack on the roof of the car. He walked a few steps toward the darkness by a tree in our neighbor's yard and proceeded to take a piss. I announced, "Hey, Kale, over here!" He slowly turned his head toward us and announced, "Yeah, be right there!"

(Kale never did show much concern for the law. I once pulled up to Rob's bar and found Kale sleeping casually in his car with his boots sticking out the window. His car was not running but it had rolled over the sidewalk and was now resting against an abandoned building with the headlights still on and a beer bottle on the roof of his car. His good times were not to be hindered by legalities.)

I would introduce him to my roommates and they proceeded to offer him some keg beer. Within an hour, Kale, myself, and several others were smoking a couple of joints I had saved in my bedroom. Joints were somewhat of a treat as we usually ended up poking holes in a beer can to make a disposable pipe. We all seemed to get along pretty well, just as people normally do while high. The party grew to be standing room only but fairly uneventful. The cops arrived as usual and proceeded to file people out the backdoor, handing out underage consumption violations. Kale and I were currently sitting in my car in the darkness of the back alley behind the house, burning the two roaches from our prior joints. I guess we figured the cops were too busy to notice us. We were not socially inept, but there seemed to be a different level of conversation among college kids and working-class people. (I came to that conclusion long ago.) And neither of us were friends with the law. So I believed we were in the safest place.

He proceeded to tell me that a few weeks ago, while on some mountain road in Idaho, he had a battle with a large stranger. Kale, a local coworker from Idaho, and this large stranger were en route to another bar in this guy's truck when Kale told him to keep his eyes on the road as they were nearing the edges of some steep overhangs. Kale was sitting in the middle. The stranger began to taunt him and his friend by swerving and acting like he was going off the road. Kale quickly grew tired of his actions.

Kale explained, "So I yanked the steering wheel to the right and said, 'Here, you wanna die, fucker? Let's do it!' I let go, and he cranked it back on the road and locked up his brakes and threw it in park. Then the big fucker grabs my neck and starts choking me! I felt fucked for a few seconds! I reached down into the twelve-pack we had on the floor and grabbed a full can of beer. I pulled it out and slammed it butt first on his forehead! I think it was the second or third hit that exploded the beer and got him off me! Beer sprayed everywhere!"

"Then what?" I replied with anticipation.

"Well, I musta dazed the fucker 'cause I heard him let out a moan, so we got out the passenger side and ran around and pulled him out his door. He was kinda fucked up, so me and Jimmy drug him to the side of the road and left him there. We took his truck to town and left it at the gas station."

"Wow!" I paused, letting the story soak in. "Whatever happened to him?"

"To who? Jimmy?"

"No. The guy you thumped."

"Oh. Never heard nothin' about it. We were gone in a couple days."

The weight of our conversation was suddenly lifted when I discovered several butts protruding from my broken car stereo as I informed Kale that the tape deck was not the ashtray.

We seemed to continue our same lifestyles over the course of the following year. Kale frequently attempted to reconcile with his ex-girlfriend and establish some form of life while still working on the road. He would return on occasion and seem to have a new story every time. He was currently working and staying with a rough kind of crowd. Apart from each other, and he made no indication to me at the time, he was also beginning to dabble with heavier drugs, as was I.

CHAPTER 8

Drugs and Alcohol

Belittled

Lucent be the drunken face
Who steals the moments from time and space.
To live to be numb and remember nothing
Be erased of the fact: you could
have been something.
Smiles with ignorance does the drunken fool
who lives but not to die
For you are not what you were
given and belittled,… so am I.

It was the summer of '91. I was still living and working in our college town and my brother kept me involved in softball and painting houses on weekends for extra cash. I had no serious girlfriends. I would meet several girls through my college friends at our party house, but it was hard to hold any conversations about what I considered to be the *real* issues in life. I often felt like an outsider in our home and found myself going back to Rob's bar when time allowed.

It was the Fourth of July. A few weeks earlier, I tried acid for the first time. I must have had the correct amount because other than noticing how pretty the lights were and how green the trees could be, I felt little else. I wasn't drinking.

Now we were at a populated lake, where there were several bars scattered around the area. I was with Kale, Dave, and a few other greaser friends of ours. Kale and these friends were on their second day of partying as they explained how they showered out in the rain the day before with soap and shampoo. Completely on my own, I managed to score a couple of squares of some kind of paper acid. It was like a miniature stamp. Just drop it in your mouth and see what happens. I took one and gave one to Kale.

I would spend most of the day drinking more beer than I thought I could ever handle. My memory is fleeting, and it wouldn't be right to put down some of the things that I thought happened as I'm not sure they did. At the time, Kale said his didn't seem to have much effect on him, but I was in the spirit world. I had some mild, yet unfriendly hallucinations and went from having fun early on to feeling crazy and sick.

Late that night, there were four of us left in the car when we found a gravel road to stop and sleep. I was still seeing some things that may or may not have been there. I asked Kale to stay awake with me. He could tell I needed company. We stayed up talking for several hours. I remember him first telling me to think happy thoughts and to remind myself that it was just the acid. Later, when I calmed down but still couldn't sleep, he told me that I was hanging with the wrong crowd, that I shouldn't be doing this to myself. He then asked the logical question "If it's not fun, why are you doing it?"

I would return to work the next day and suffer one of the worst hangovers on record. It was the last acid trip I'd ever taken.

"Dudes on ludes should not drive!"

Late that summer, Kale and I were hanging out at Rob's bar when we were offered Valium. It is just a widely prescribed anti-anxiety, sleeping pill. That is basically what it does to you. I found it to be a great remedy for my overanxious mind. It's known as a downer, and as bad as it sounds, it really is just anti-anxiety medication. But just like all medications, it's not to be taken with alcohol.

Kale had signed up to begin lineman school in a bordering state starting in the fall. He had already begun reading several textbooks he acquired from a relative. He was driving a late-seventies, early-eighties maroon Dodge Diplomat. ("She rides five but only sleeps four!") It had seen its share of hard times.

It was a Sunday afternoon. Feeling a slight hangover from the night before, a friend handed us each two Valium blues. Kale immediately put his in his pocket and disappeared. Still sitting next to the guy who gave them to us, I asked how powerful they are. He recommended that I bite one in half and see how that does. Kale returned a couple of minutes later.

Innocently, he asked, "Hey, you take yours yet?"

"No. He told me to take half of one to see what it does."

Looking at the 'dealer', Kale said, "What the fuck? Are they pretty strong?"

"Well, I wouldn't take 'em both at the same time. Did you?" he asked.

Kale replied, "Yeah! Shit! How much time do I have before they kick in?"

"About ten to fifteen minutes," he answered.

"All right, I'm outta here!"

I wouldn't hear about the rest of his adventure until a couple of weeks later.

"Hey, what happened that Sunday we took Valium?" I asked.

"Oh, I got busted goin' home!" Kale responded. (He was currently staying with his mother, Joan, about thirty miles away from Rob's bar.) "It's all in the police report, if you want to see it!"

"Give me your version," I replied.

"Well, my piece-of-shit car is somewhat responsible. I musta been lookin' at the power line poles, ya know, thinkin', *That's a b-phase. That's a transmission line.* Then, when I look back at the road, I'm in the fuckin' ditch! I was only goin' about twenty miles an hour, but I couldn't keep the bitch on the road! Fuckin' drugs!"

"Well, how'd the cop find ya?" I asked.

"Well, apparently, there was an old couple at an intersection who called the cops, sayin' I was in the ditch. They said they had to back up so I could drive across the approach in front of them. I already had a flat tire at the time!"

Concerned, but laughing, I said, "Go on."

"So I'm limpin' this piece o' shit through town when the cop pulls me over. Now I blow another tire, pullin' over 'cause o' fuckin rebar stickin' out where they're redoin' the sidewalk! I step outta the car, and the cops walks up and says, 'Just what the fuck you think you're doin?' I point at the car and say, 'You try drivin' that son of a bitch! That fuckin' thing ain't fit for the road!' So the cop says, 'Well, what are you doin' drivin it?' I told him, 'Well, I had to get home!'"

Laughing, I replied, "You gotta be shittin' me!"

"No. I wish I was. I saw it all in the police report. I guess I went on to tell him about my vise grip holdin' the brake line on, and when you hit the brake, you go in *this* ditch, when you let off, you go *that* ditch! Ha-ha! Yeah, he was pissed, but I remember him laughin' when he was tellin' his partner."

"Did you get a DWI?" I asked.

"No. I blew a 0.08! [DWIs were 0.10 at this time.] Yeah, they kept lookin' at me when they were takin' my blood at the hospital like 'What the fuck is wrong with this guy?'"

"So you didn't get anything?"

"Naw. Well, they gave me an exhibition driving ticket. S'pose to go to court next month."

(Later, he would tell this story to his ex-girlfriend Rachel. Because of an argument they'd recently had, she sent a letter to the police, informing them of his admittance to taking Valium. They would then try to reinstate a DWI charge. Through his lawyer, I believe they later settled on a reckless driving charge.)

Later that summer, in another act of experimentation, or maybe a subconscious search for this thing that I seemed to be lacking, I would try cocaine. Kale was not around. At this point in my life, I was possibly still easily influenced. I was not just fearless—I was oblivious to fear. My coworkers and I drank almost every night, and I was either partying or recovering from partying. In this consistent, confusing state of mind, there was little time for contemplating serious decisions.

But here I was, with a few acquaintances that I wouldn't now consider my friends and several strangers, drinking at a small-town bar. We ended up at an after-bar party, and before I was aware of it, I was snorting a line. Through the drunken haze, I remember a feeling that I'd never had before. Inhibitions and my usual lack of confidence were completely absent within minutes. It was the beginning of a two-day bender, and where we went, what we did, and who I was with are all but lost from memory. We drank continuously, and there are moments of memory that include other bars, a restaurant, and a sight that burned itself into my memory. At some point, I recall seeing two guys laid back on a couch, completely incoherent. One had a needle still dangling from his arm. The host, noticing this, quickly escorted us to another room. I knew I was in a setting I had never been before, and I knew that I didn't belong. It still wasn't enough to scare me back into consciousness because late Sunday night, someone had to remind me that on Monday, I had a job. We just couldn't continue to do this.

Everything I'd ever heard about coke was true. There is absolutely no way to be depressed while on it. *Euphoric* is an understatement. And the things you will do and say to continue this feeling are inconceivable. Fortunately, it was gone. And I didn't seem to know anyone well enough to keep it coming. It was obvious that an electrician's wages couldn't keep this habit going for more than a weekend.

Kale enrolled in lineman school that fall. I would inform him of my coke adventure. He replied, "Yeah. I did it before. All I remember is being at a gas station filling up my car, thinkin' to myself, 'I'm the coolest fucker in the world that ever put gas in a car!' That shit is amazing! Hard to quit though. Ain't it, Johnny?"

"Damn straight!" I replied. "Best to leave that shit alone!"

Kale would return from school on occasion and was feeling really good about his grades and his new line of work ahead of him. We were standing outside Rob's. Calling me a 'narrow back' (a lineman's term for electrician), Kale convinced me to try to climb the power pole in front of the bar using his gaffs. I was gullible. Having never attempted this before, about halfway up, I noticed my feet wanting to slide out of the gaffs. I complained to Kale.

Looking up, Kale said, "Yeah, you should be wearing work boots with heels."

"You mean I shouldn't be doin' this wearing my tennis shoes?"

Laughing, he replied, "Well, you can, but they don't recommend it!"

I managed to climb back down. Kale put on the gear and quickly climbed to the top like a squirrel. Sitting at the top, he told me to throw him a beer. In awe of this new skill, I refused. Pulling out a smoke and proud as a peacock, he exclaimed, "I like it better up here than I do on the ground, Johnny!" He went on to tell me that in school, they often climbed to the top and played catch with a basketball pole to pole. He said that about half the class quit at this point.

I would visit Kale at his school. I was working about an hour away from him. He wasn't drinking much at all. He was studying and liking it. He wanted me to learn chess. He said his roommate taught him a few weeks ago and that he hadn't been beaten since. I told him that I didn't have the time or patience to learn chess right now.

"Ahh, c'mon! It's easy!"

I wanted to go out and hit the bars. He said he didn't have the money and that it was not as much fun here as I would think it is. So we shared that undeniable, somewhat uncomfortable feeling you get when one of your friends decides to quit drinking and you don't know how to act around each other. And it was what we'd done together for years, so I did notice it. Kale didn't try to convince me not to drink. He just said he was taking a break. Other than physical feats or maybe forcing me to stand up for myself, he'd never intentionally persuaded me to do anything in my life. And I certainly couldn't persuade him to do anything—up to this point, I don't know if I ever have. But it was a Saturday night. I hadn't skipped drinking on a Saturday night since I had the flu. I wish he would've used his unintentional influence on me to get me to join him in his sobriety.

These were Kale's good days. He had a spring in his step again—literally; he used his whole foot when he walked, extending off his toes. Simple things became fun again. He was outgoing and more social. He seemed to drink less and laugh more. And he had always had a loud, genuine laugh. When we did party, he danced like no one was watching, and he was well aware that he sucked at it. What people call cutting a rug, he called 'slicin' the carpet' as he acted it out like he was actually slicing carpet with his boots. There was still no undiscussed 'elephant in the room' in his presence, but he was using more tact. He hadn't been in a fight for some time. He was broke but needed little. He was getting along well with his friends and family as his sister was recently married and had a baby girl.

Kale had never been what I consider an asshole. He'd always been the first guy to open doors for strangers, pick up hitchhikers, and help stranded motorists. He was well aware that it felt good to do good. He was also making a few new friends at school and was enjoying the learning process. This was why we were friends. This was how I had hoped life would continue.

Life was good for Kale and his family. Kale's brother Steve would begin working for Dan, our mutual childhood friend, building substations around the Midwest. Kale would continue with lineman school. Life was good for all of us. I was about to embark on this world-renowned insanity called 'love'.

CHAPTER 9

Kacey

Yesterday, I had to play electrician again. Couldn't write. Today? Sucked. Noticed how it felt like depression, but was just like the more 'human' version of being in a bad mood. Couldn't create. Allergic to electrical work or maybe I was under the false impression that becoming a 'writer' would end my misery. Still sober so I can't blame booze. Writing is not like any other job; cannot just force it. Have to wait for the right mood. Have to find balance.

—January 24, 2014, daily
journal (unedited)

Beautiful Things

The attractions will vary, but the results are the
same.
We're drawn to the danger like moths to the
flame.
Superficial smiles will bring you to your knees;
This unobtainable beauty, yet I still believe.
A lifetime of yearning and the frustration it brings
In the endless pursuit of beautiful things.

It was the Fourth of July weekend in 1992. We met by random chance. There had been no arrangement, unless by God. Kacey was dressed rather conservatively, like going out was unexpected. Her brown eyes and flawless face were slightly covered by her brown shoulder-length hair. I sensed no makeup as it was unnecessary. She was wearing a light jacket, likely not her own, which was always necessary at our summertime street dances. She stood around 5 feet seven inches; a tall and slender look with curves in all the right places. I know she was beautiful from head to toe, but I couldn't take my eyes off her legs, although I'd claim that I was not superficial. The faded and ageless 'Daisy Dukes' shorts accentuated a perfectly tanned skin tone, which only looks natural on certain people. It was as if she was the Caucasian version of the Pocahontas fantasies I had since puberty.

I had a removable walking cast on my leg from a sprained knee I acquired playing softball the weekend prior. I managed to drive myself there and was now using crutches to get around. I was portrayed as harmless and approachable and played the part well.

It was a fairly slow night for a dance and I was slow to drink as I had to wait for a friend to bring me a beer. I found her sitting on the same set of bleacher seats alone for a moment, so I slid (slithered) a little closer. (Boy, do I miss self-confidence.) We exchanged small talk for a few seconds when I discovered she was a friend of my friend's girlfriend Becky. (Odds are, I was going to know someone.) Upon witnessing our conversation, this boisterous girlfriend, Becky, quickly approached to tell me, "Back off, Johnny, this one is engaged!" Playing the role of the self-centered womanizer I likely may have been at the time, I responded toward Kacey, "You can't get married! You haven't had me yet."

This would set the tone for the good-humored, yet assertive dialogue between us. I knew this was not her first time responding to pick-up lines. Girls who look like her have to be used to it. I now laid it on fairly thick because I didn't seem to fear rejection if I'd assume it was coming. So by instantly considering her unattainable, I was free to be loose and somewhat arrogant, which ironically, is quite becoming to girls. (Go figure.)

Kasey was not old enough to drink, eighteen, so I don't think she did, certainly not enough to be drunk and not in public anyway. She found herself playing defense most of the night as it became humorous while I made such comments as "We're gonna have beautiful children" and "Don't laugh. I'll change your name someday."

As the night went on, I believe Becky suggested we all meet at a house party en route to her home. I somehow managed to convince Kacey to ride with me. We wouldn't make it. (This is the age before cell phones, and it was very easy to get yourself lost.) After an hour of driving around our local gravel farm roads, sipping on a beer, we arrived at my parents' home.

I was now twenty-two years old, three and half years older than Kacey. I was likely telling her that she was too young to know what she wanted to do with her life (like I knew). I learned that she was enrolled at the same college as her fiancé, who happened to be the quarterback, but I quickly changed that subject. I had yet to kiss her as I truly believed she wouldn't let me. I had been in this position several times, and my astute awareness was centered on gauging the opposite sex's reactive body language. And it was telling me I was not getting any, but I was truly enjoying our conversation. We had been talking for hours. She continued to show some interest, but it was now closer to sunrise than darkness. I told her I had to get my injured knee elevated as I crawled into bed. She reluctantly joined me but kept blankets between us to try and create somewhat of a sexual barrier. Cautious, hesitant, and nearing sobriety now, I thought of the many consequences. I had a girlfriend of a couple months who was starting to really like me, and I made the mistake of letting her, knowing she was not the one. She would be hurt. Kacey was engaged to be married, and he was a college quarterback, and quarterbacks would always have huge friends who serve and protect them. These thoughts that would usually save you from collateral damage were instantly obliterated the moment our lips finally met. The blanket barrier would fail.

My friends had always perceived me as someone who took lightly these encounters and I found it easier to pretend to be that guy instead of explaining the truth: that I was just a human being unconsciously and consciously in search of a mate, and that although I was very particular for love, I would try many, yet I would not love many, but I would love deeply.

I'm definitely not a stranger to meaningless one-night stands and have had several before my last girlfriend. (There is such a thing as a one-night stand, but if you pay attention, you'll find it usually means something, and eventually, it can define you.) The next day, I told myself that this was all that it was; I just got extremely lucky one night. She'd go back to the quarterback, marry, have children, and live a happy life, and carry with her a secret one-night stand with a fast-talking townie. I would use this night as a high watermark and to build confidence for when the right one would come along. But there was no time.

To my surprise, I received a phone call the next afternoon. It was from a younger sister of an ex-girlfriend I dated in high school. We knew each other well but rarely spoke on the phone. It turned out she was also a friend of Kacey's and asked me if I'd like to meet up with the two of them later that night.

The three of us arrived at yet another street dance. (What else?) Kacey was now made up. Her Daisy Dukes were accompanied by a long-sleeve bright-white top with ruffles down the front, accentuating her perfect skin tone. Her hair seemed magically longer, done by whatever girls do to make that possible. I truly believed that at this moment, there was no man alive who could say no to her. Our mutual friend left us within an hour of our arrival.

We walked. I was still in my cast but without crutches now and managed fairly well as we made our way down the main street. Her beauty was unmatched in this small town, and we got double and triple takes everywhere we went. Some guys were likely contemplating injuring themselves just be in my shoes. We recognized some friends of ours at different places, and I enjoyed the interactions. Kacey seemed confident, yet insecure at the right moments, enough to keep her real and put me more at ease. We seemed more concerned with what we said to each other than our conversations with friends, so they tended to quickly leave us.

Now in seclusion, for some reason, I began to reveal some of my past. I told her that my reputation was far worse than who I was. I told her that I'd been in trouble with the law often in my past. I told her that three years ago in this same town, I picked up a girl, and we went home together. I told her how I was charged with rape and that I narrowly escaped spending the better half of my life behind bars.

Kacey didn't seem too concerned with this, like she already knew. She was a very good listener; she empathized well.

As we continued, likely feeling obligated to also reveal something from her past, she disclosed to me that while she was spending the summer in the city, she was a nanny for a wealthy couple. Some stripper friends she met while doing this convinced her to show up at their strip club for amateur night. She did, and she won. Taking home over two thousand dollars that night, she returned a couple of times to see if she could make that much again. She found that it wasn't as profitable as she first thought and gave it up. In an attempt to bring light to the depth of this conversation, I proclaimed, "So we're just a stripper and a rapist walkin' the street. Sounds about right." Again, I would somehow convince her to accompany me home.

It was only my second night with Kacey. We slept in contact, like intertwined snakes seeking warmth, as if we'd been waiting a long time to meet. There was an obvious instant connection being made as we were together, selfishly in our own world. Neither one of us was going to ruin this by speaking too much of the past or by bringing up questions of the future. This moment would not be wagered.

On day 3; it was a Sunday. My brother picked me up about noon to complete a paint job on a barn. I had mentioned to Kacey the night before that I had to work and where the job was located. Midway through the day, Kacey and our mutual friend arrived at the jobsite. They hung around for a while. Before they left, I informed Kacey that I would be heading to my day job later that day. I told her I would stop to see her at our friend's home who also lived in the area.

Within an hour after my arrival, I got the feeling that Kacey was likely homeless after her weekend escapade. (Her parents currently lived in the city, over three hours away.) Or if she failed to mention any of this to her fiancé, she would likely be homeless soon. I told her that my boss had an apartment rented for me and a few coworkers near our jobsite, which was about two hours away. Other than that, I had been intermittently living with my parents on the weekends. Feeling somewhat responsible for her dilemma, and still very much wanting her in my presence, I invited her to stay with me on the road for the week.

Convinced I won't be killed, I brought her to meet her fiancé so she could pick up a few things. She had him believing that she needed time to think about her future and that I was just a long-time friend of the family who was willing to give her a ride to her aunt's home on my way to work. Yeah, she was very convincing. Very polite and cordial, he thanked me for helping her out. Surprised and relieved, we continued on our way.

Before the week was up, our Bonnie-and-Clyde adventure was over. Her parents and her fiancé had been in touch and evidently made several phone calls trying to locate her, including one to my boss. Being the upstanding citizen he pretended to be, he then contacted me and threatened to fire me if she showed up the following week. We decided to cut ties for a while.

A couple of days after meeting Kacey, I did one thing right: I told my prior girlfriend that she deserved better than me. That, apparently, I was not mature enough to have a girlfriend. It was a short relationship, but I shouldn't have let her believe it had a future. Karma would arrive soon.

Whatever deep, sincere thoughts of a future relationship most people should have at a time like this were somewhere lost from consciousness. You simply couldn't ask me to be logical, discerning, or reasonable while in Kacey's presence. I should see this as dangerous. But I don't. I dropped off Kacey at her friend's home and we parted ways. Although she embedded herself deep inside my mind, it didn't last long enough to call myself heartbroken… yet.

"When love is not madness, it is not love."
(Pedro Calderon de la Barcia).

My job on the road reached completion. I would continue with work back in college town. Kacey would magically reappear within weeks. The conditions surrounding how and where are beyond my recollection, but she was abruptly back in my life. Both of us were currently indifferent to consequence. She would meet my friends and family. They were all very impressed. She was charming, charismatic, social, and very attentive to me. There was no sign of misrepresentation. Even Kale's incisive ability to spot a phony was sidetracked. (I always asked his opinion.) He said nothing, not because he didn't notice, but because she was real. Being beautiful and brilliant, Kacey would rule my world. My rarely sober, oversexed mind saw nothing but bliss.

We were staying in my parents' basement but began to search for our own place. I was still living paycheck to paycheck and finding a cheap apartment was difficult. Kacey was not working and seemed to evade the subject every time I brought it up. She believed that the only way to get a fresh start and get ahead of our situation was for her to return to the city, dance for a couple weeks, and possibly make upward of about four thousand dollars. I argued with obvious reasoning. She explained that there was a difference in strippers. There were those who were willing to do anything for money, and then there were those who were professional and respectable; the type that truly were paying their own way through college. Personally, I had only been to see strippers once in my life at this point and obtained nowhere near enough knowledge to form an opinion. It wouldn't have mattered. As naive and easily manipulated as I was, and as convincing as Kacey could be, I released her to the city in my father's car. She was to return in two weeks.

She called upon her arrival and gave me her work phone number and the number to her friend's home where she was staying. I left her alone for the most part and tried to distract myself with other projects until this would pass. It was definitely not something you'd brag about to your friends, so I wasn't very sociable. Although I did hang out with Kale and his brother Steve. There never had been anything going on in my life that I didn't share with them.

The two weeks went by and Kacey didn't return. I called to find out why and was given many excuses, with the most believable one being that the club was holding her money because she owed them from the last time she was there. I was beginning to realize that she was likely gone, but my father was still missing his car. Kacey now hung up on me when I asked for the car over the next couple of days. On Sunday, I took the spare keys and convinced Kale's brother Steve to drive me the two hundred miles to the club.

We arrive in Steve's '69 Charger RT. I checked the parking lot for the Olds Delta 98—nothing. I walked inside expecting some serious drama. I could get beaten and thrown out, arrested, or shot, and the least would be to have to witness my girlfriend on stage. Steve told me to just be cool. "We're here to get a car."

It was completely uneventful. We didn't find Kacey or the car. I did recognize the name of one of her friends at the club, the only thing that made this seem real. I explained the situation and told her to tell Kacey that if the car wasn't back in two days, it would be reported as stolen. We left unscathed.

Kacey called me the next day, seemingly unaffected. "Sorry, I'll bring it back tomorrow night. I'll meet you at your parents' house." She hung up before I could speak.

I wait. No car. No Kacey. I called our mutual friend Becky at our nearby college town and asked her if she could drive around to see if she could find the car in the chance that Kacey parked it somewhere near her so as to avoid a confrontation with me. She called back to inform me that she found it parked near my boss's shop and that it'd been damaged.

I arrived to see that there was a considerable amount of body damage done to it. I brought it home to my father with my tail between my legs. I agreed to pay for it to be repaired.

The very next weekend, I called the club. To my surprise, they put her on the phone. Trying hard to stay calm, I said, "What the fuck was that? You wrecked my dad's car! You're goddamn lucky you're not in jail!"

In an unrecognizable voice, she responded loud enough for her friends to hear, "Whew, my man's pissed!"

Then, as if she wanted me to know, I literally heard the sound of her snorting a line. Having had the experience, I heard the long inhale, the shortened exhaling grunts, right down to the tapping on the glass to reform the next line. I subconsciously wished I had some. Not knowing what to do next, I followed in the footsteps of the last guy in my position and reluctantly called her mother.

Kacey's parents were middle-class, fairly successful people. I understood them to be very concerned parents, judging by Kacey's respect for them. I had only spoken to them a couple of times up to this point, but I felt I had to inform them of what just transpired. (I'd like to think I did this for her as an act of kindness. But even kindness can be selfish.)

This was the part where my belief in doing the right thing just happened to coincide with my own insecurities and my inability to just let her go. I begin playing the martyr—I would suffer for the cause.

Several hours later, I got a call. Kacey and her mother were on both phones at their home and arguing with me over what had just transpired. Apparently, her parents managed to retrieve her from the club. Kacey was denying anything and everything. Her speech was pressured and hurried but very articulate, and when she got done chewing my ass, I questioned myself and what it was I did hear. (It was what she did best.) She told her mother to get off the phone.

Kacey and I continued our conversation. Beginning to cry, she told me that she was fucked up, that she needed help, and that her parents wanted to send her somewhere. I told her to go. "Please go." I made her no promises, but she complied. I secretly felt a good sensation before sleeping that night . . . and it was selfish.

> Doormat;
> A figment of my imagination is worded;
> I write to achieve, though it devours my strength.
> I find words to express a feeling of doubt,
> On the canvass of a doormat.

Kacey called from rehab. Her voice was shallow and calm and sweet. "They tell me I can have visitors. Would you like to come and see me?" With little hesitation, I complied.

It was a beautiful fall day. I was accompanied by my brother. Kacey was wearing a gold blazer that made her look professional, like a Century 21 agent. My brother made a wise comment about it. (It was what he did best.) The three of us had a smoke on a park bench. Treating it like a drunken weekend, my brother looked at Kacey and inquired with a smile, "So ... did you have a good time?"

Taking it in stride, Kacey responded, "Well, judging from my position, I must have."

After exchanging some lighthearted small talk, my brother left us to talk. I made every inquiry I dreamed up in the last couple of weeks. I wanted every possible reason for her actions. I wanted her to explain to me how she could do this. I wanted her to give me something to hate because I'd never hate her.

She told me they found traces of drugs in her system, but no cocaine (I would eventually learn that cocaine can be quickly and naturally dispersed from your system). I asked her what the hell was going up her nose when she was on the phone with me—as if being addicted to coke would be a sufficient explanation. She said she didn't know, that the whole event was blurry and hard to remember.

She teared up while apologizing for the car and informed me to tell my dad that she'd pay for the damage. As if I knew what I was talking about, I told her not to worry about that, to just get well, to take this time seriously. I heard the words "I'm sorry" again. I made no promises out loud, and we shared a long hug. She walked away hiding her tears.

Later, through phone calls, Kacey would reveal secrets to me, secrets about her past. Secrets that, although they did not involve her family, if you heard them, you would not doubt their validity. But I didn't want to feel sorry for her. I wanted to love her. Telling me these childhood secrets had me believe that she now trusted me and that she was truly sorry. That as long as we understood each other and trust each other, this was still going to work.

Kacey would move back in with her parents in the city. During the next couple of weeks, we spoke frequently on the phone. She convinced me to meet her parents in person.

On the way, I contemplated my future. I knew that I loved her, from what I know of love, yet something was seriously wrong. I had now been detached for a couple of weeks and was beginning to finally hear the advice from my close friends and family. I had to leave her. If she was to ever get better, she could only do so without me. I had already broken the rule—that how-to-stay-safe rule: never love someone more than they love you. This was going to cost me.

I should run away. I shouldn't look back. But in the way that only psychology even comes close to defining, I was not going anywhere. I seemed to associate my happiness with her. I may just be too young and too arrogant to believe that I could be hurt. Completely disregarding the risks, I only saw what I wanted to see—that she did drugs, that she wasn't herself, and that she loved me and was going to do everything necessary to make it work with me—and I couldn't allow myself to be wrong about that.

I would officially meet her family. Kacey was the oldest of three girls. Her parents were young, late thirties, attractive, intelligent, and successful people. They were very kind to me and seemed relieved to know I was not as bad as they likely predicted. I was involved, yet I was trying to find a way to excuse myself. When they inquired about our future, hoping that leaving her could actually become a reality to me by verbalizing, I told them that I couldn't do this anymore and that I had to get my life back in order. I later had a talk with Kacey about this, but when I left, I left the door open. I again told Kacey that I was a phone call away if she needed to talk. I left relieved and sad but still under her spell.

I returned to my parents' basement. Kacey began to appear out of nowhere, sometimes at 4:00 a.m., rarely explaining herself. Her parents' home was at least two hundred miles away. Sometimes she wouldn't even wake me. She would just be there when I woke up, sleeping next to me in the crook of my arm, looking even more beautiful than when she was awake. I would often leave her sleeping while I got up and left for work.

What most healthy people don't understand is that this behavior builds strong bonds between unhealthy people. Well, at least it did for me. I didn't recognize the unhealthy behavior. I recognized the desire to be necessary. I didn't think I'd ever had this much use for myself. In psychological terms, this was obviously a codependent, symbiotic, dysfunctional relationship. In laymen's terms, the rocks in my head matched the holes in her's.

Within a couple of weeks, I was still not seeing clearly. Kacey had obviously been upsetting her parents by taking their car without permission and not complying with their rules at home. She was nineteen now. She was not under house arrest. She could leave at any time. I would like to say I was persuaded, but I did it on my own. I made the drive to the city and stole her away.

We were broke. Problems were right around the corner. We found a one-bedroom apartment, and I took what furniture was unused from my parents' home. Silverware was not on my list as I remember having to share a fork for a couple days while we ate. (How romantic.)

There was still nothing normal about our relationship. I knew nothing about her daily life. If I went out with coworkers after work, she wouldn't be home when I got there. We continued to fight about everyday issues, with money being a major concern. I confronted her regularly about a job. She lied. I never knew where she was or what she was doing, and our time together was spent arguing, making insecure accusations, and aggressively defending ourselves.

I again make yet another idle threat. I told her something that neither she nor I believed: that I was not going to live this way, that I was done. There was no way I could tolerate this behavior. My anxiety-ridden and depressed mind had already based my happiness upon her, but the laws of self-preservation were at the forefront. I was close to losing what was left of my mind. I had to move on. There was no way I could prepare for such a life. (But it would seem that the spirit of an unborn child would prove persistent.)

Her parents and I would convince her to move back with her family in the city.

We went through the motions of a normal couple breaking up. We began to separate the few things we shared together—she got the spoon while I got the fork. I was not positive she'd move back with her parents, so I didn't ask where she'd live or what she'd do. I cared deeply, and I was trying hard not to, so I was likely drunk.

I was depressed. I looked around the apartment and all I saw was her. I never noticed anything else in the room when Kacey was here. I told myself that I'd get better, but I drank alone now. I was still trying hard to be somebody—an alcoholic maybe? That was someone.

A couple of weeks later, Kacey called from her parents' home. She behaved like we didn't just break up, and according to my actions, it was the appropriate response. She complained of having to work odd hours at a mall and spend a lot of time riding busses to and from work. I was not sympathetic, but when she spoke of how much she missed me, she cried or sat in silence, sobbing. I was not equipped to handle distant empathy.

I brought her back within the month. We celebrated our insanity and went back to the same routine. It was now November. I'd known her less than six months.

> Being used
> It's a feeling of loss that I can't explain
> The empty stare from her face; is she the cause
>   of my pain?
> Wanting her to stay while she walks away
> If I slap her face, will my pain go away?
> Lust from her touch has led me confused
> Pretending I don't know that I'm being used.

When we fought, she left. I suffered without her, yet she always managed to show up before I could 'get right'. We took turns seeking each other out. When I pursued her, she eluded. When I gave up, she returned. I was obviously lacking the self-esteem necessary or the sobriety required to commit to saying no to her and leaving her alone. She showed up on occasion, unannounced at any hour, and I took her in every time. (The Offspring's "Self-Esteem" song comes to mind.) I was surprised every time I saw her, yet I was beside myself when I didn't know where she was. She was better at hiding than I was, and better at leaving. But sometimes she showed up drunk and crying. Other times, she seemed fine, and we contemplated a future together.

In December, we found out we were pregnant. It was not something I was going to shout from the rooftops. Part of me thought, *Finally, she'll settle down—not me, her.* We moved into a two-bedroom apartment on the other side of town. Kacey took a job at a local tanning salon. Now completely sober, she was becoming the person that I always thought she could be: responsible, caring, attentive, and very lovable.

It was a happier time in my life. I felt lucky. Our past seemed to be essentially forgotten. We became closer with each other's families (mine knew little of our recent past.)

Kacey carried a baby well. According to our friends, she could model maternity clothes with her pregnant look, and I was still very attracted to her. When we went out together, we caught each other ignoring our friends and sharing looks from across the room. This was real. It seemed we have temporarily gotten past the chaos of our childish ways.

I was very much in love. Why wouldn't I be? She was not going anywhere now. I got to do the things I did before and quickly returned to them. I drank. I smoked. I stay out late, with or without her. I hadn't changed much at all. I was still the person I used to be: selfish, immature, and rarely home. Even at twenty-three years old, my hangovers and unacknowledged depression caused me to become isolated and emotionally detached. She was likely lonely even when I was there.

I also had way too many friends. They formed my identity. I loved and craved their attention. When Kale was in the area, I dropped any responsibilities and spent my free time with him, so much so that even Kale often told me to go home. I tended to put all my friends above my girlfriend and unborn child. She was sober now, and it was not a matter of whether or not she was deserving; it had become obvious—I only knew how to behave when I was about to lose her.

CHAPTER 10

Thomas and a Brief Marriage

Hear the cries of the lonely child, who dreams attention's love of smiles. He waits for the hands of gentle grace, the whisper of love, the smile of face.

— "Smile of Face"

I turned twenty-three in February of '93. I was a good man. As long I got to do whatever I wanted and within the positive realm of my friends' and family's approval, I would be good to my girlfriend. I was forewarned by my brother about the mood swings of pregnant women and told to tend to their strange needs as best I could. If she desired chicken strips at 2:00 a.m., I'd go get chicken strips! She'd likely be sleeping when I'd return, but she'd appreciate the effort. From my understanding, Kacey's mood swings were not much different than a bad menstrual cycle. Anything short of our first few months together was a blessing to me.

Although she was likely harboring some anger toward my behavior, we had become a seemingly normal couple — smitten; accidentally calling each other honey and finishing each other's sentences. We were looking forward to having a baby, as was our families.

My son, Thomas, was brought into the world on July 20. I witnessed the chaos of his birth. He entered upside down and pissed off! I had no idea he held the power to sustain another's life.

Kale arrived that night to celebrate with me. He agreed to have one beer with me. He was on the wagon at the time, so he drove while we barhopped and I passed out cigars. He had recently graduated lineman school and was to begin working with his brother Steve and our friend Dan, building substations. He was in a very good place.

At home, my socializing was soon cut in half. Kacey proved to be a good mother for a twenty-year-old, considering neither of us have had any experience at self-discipline. Her being the eldest sibling in her family, she may have acquired some knowledge of infants, but mine was nonexistent. I had a niece and a nephew at the time, and as much as I loved to make them smile, until they could interact with me, babies were just an eating, pooping, crying machine. I was selfish this way.

It wasn't long before I returned to my self-centered ways. I again became the man that often came home at 2:00 a.m., drunk, sometimes stoned, cooked a pizza, and watched *Beavis and Butthead*. If I had a friend with me, too drunk to continue driving, he'd sleep on our couch. All these things were the norm before Thomas was born. And I was slow to change.

I remember a fully-packed, duffel bag sitting in front of the door to our apartment one night. Kale was with me. It had a note on it that read something like this: "If you choose to open the door and come in, you are choosing to quit partying all night, you are choosing to pay more attention to me and your son, and you are giving up your fucked-up lifestyle. Think it through. You can come and get the rest of your shit tomorrow. I'm not doing this anymore. Love, Kacey."

I chose to walk in. I convinced Kale to stay, but he wisely left early in the morning.

Unlike my prior idle threats, Kacey rarely gave ultimatums. I reluctantly did what I was asked, but only for as long as I thought necessary.

Amanda

Kacey had also acquired a new friend— Amanda. She was short, round, energetic, and a pleasure to be around. Her son was older than Thomas, but they seemed to keep each other entertained. Kacey now went out with Amanda on occasion. I stayed home with Thomas. Considering my lifestyle, it seemed a fair trade-off at first. I didn't ask questions or complain. I likely had some of this coming.

I believe we were out shopping for groceries. Kacey thought it was time we should look at rings. I took it as a proposal. I didn't refuse. Before we could have a serious conversation about it, the date was set for July the following year.

Months would pass, and they must have been fairly uneventful as I only chose to remember the negative. The hype created making wedding plans superseded the actual thought of marriage. (I assume this happens often.) I got to have a bachelor party, with all my friends getting together over me. This was what I thought about.

The bachelor party—the wedding celebration for dudes. Everyone I associated with was there: my acquaintances made during city league basketball, my stoner friends, my father and his friends, to the closest of my childhood friends. It was quite an assortment. I believe it was my hometown's first and possibly last lingerie show. They likely made a new city ordinance afterward.

I behaved. I was not and never was the cheating type, although my reputation was the opposite. The truth was, I got around when single, but I usually left the girl before conversations about a relationship were started. I did respect the hearts of others. If I suspected you were beginning to feel something and I wasn't, I was usually gone. And I don't recall Kacey ever being jealous of me sexually. I gave her no reason to be. My sexual desires were fulfilled at home, and I don't recall being sexually attracted to anyone else since Kacey entered my life. She only needed more of my time and my mind.

The Thursday night before our Saturday wedding, I was drinking with my friends who were back in town for this occasion. We drove away for 'intermission'. Normally we just smoked a bowl (weed), but tonight, someone brought nose candy. I witnessed a few of them snort a line and managed to talk them out of a small amount. Kale stared at me while I formed a very small line out of the remaining coke as he asked, "You know what the fuck you're doin'? You're getting married, man!"

"I'm aware!" I replied. "This is likely the last time I ever get to do this. Don't be a dick!"

I was now in my hometown bar. I felt like the center of attention. I was marrying a beautiful and intelligent woman. I had a beautiful, healthy one-year-old son. I enjoyed the weight of the world being temporarily lifted as I hung out with all the close friends I had formed in my twenty-four years. This was my sanctuary—an hour later, reality.

It was apparent that there was no more coke. I didn't like to ever leave a bar before anyone else did, but I went to my parents' home, where my future wife and child were staying. The rehearsal is tomorrow.

When rehearsal dinner was done, Kacey was ready to go home, but I was not. We drove away together, but I told her I was coming back. She pleaded with me about the significance of the next day. "We are getting married tomorrow." I told her that after tomorrow, I wouldn't be able to see my friends as much and would like another night with all of them together. I told her that tomorrow and every day after would be about her. I was persistent and aggressively extending beyond my normal behavior, and I now know why. Even though I knew my friends had no more coke, I subconsciously wanted to be with them in case of a miracle. That was the power coke held over me. My father was also trying to convince me to go home, but I was not to be deterred. I behaved toward them in ways that I would always regret—nothing drastic, just not me.

The Wedding

Kacey looked as beautiful as expected. My friends made references to Cindy Crawford and Julia Roberts. I thought she put them to shame, but I likely didn't tell her this. My one-year-old son Thomas was the adorable ring bearer. My brother was the best man. Kale was a groomsman.

I had my doubts right up until the time we said "I do." I was not a serious religious man at the time, but I was always open to the feeling that I was doing the right thing. The groom was to wait in a room at the front of the church, out of sight, while guests were being seated. The room had a door leading outside, with the large cross standing straight up in front of you when you walk out. As I waited for my signal to re-enter, I stared up at the cross, expecting my face to smile upon receiving a feeling of approval. It didn't come. Feeling he doesn't approve, I would begin to bargain with my thoughts. "I'll be a good father if this doesn't work out. She'll be a good mother. This has to happen."

I had always had a sense of impending doom; it was in my nature. I could usually ignore it when possible and at this point in my life, I've had plenty of distractions; although it was hard to disregard these issues while staring at the cross.

The wedding dance was held outside the bar (yeah, a street dance). Our honeymoon was to take place starting Monday, so we hosted an after-bar get-together in college town at our apartment after the dance. Kacey fell asleep in a recliner. Kale ended up in our bed, so I slept on the floor. We opened gifts the following morning in my parents' backyard. My hangover-induced depression was evident. (It was recognizable in the pictures).

Monday, we left Thomas with Kacey's parents and headed for Arizona. Why Arizona in the summertime? We were there last winter to celebrate Kacey's grandmother's wedding and contemplated moving there. I was currently unemployed but had another electrician job waiting for me in college town. I wanted to see what was possible. Kacey was looking into transferring her college credits to ASU.

We held about three thousand dollars in our pocket, mostly gifts from her side. As we drove by a well-known mental health facility about an hour into our trip, I made the comment, "We should take this money and check ourselves in for the week. Maybe get a fresh start on our new life." Kacey didn't see the humor. I wasn't really kidding. I had often talked about how we could use some help. Not having a clue as to what was wrong with me at the time, I was likely trying to persuade Kacey to go.

Several hours into the trip, I noticed how quiet Kacey was, and I asked her if everything was okay. She assured me she was fine but offered nothing to the conversation. I was just realizing this was the first time we have ever spent this much time alone together without interruption or with some type of controversy to discuss since we'd known each other. If both of us were in a state of depression, we were in for a long, silent ride.

Our first stop was to see Kale. He was currently working in Colorado and renting a room in someone's home. He agreed to put us up for the night. We had a couple of beers together, but Kacey seemed exhausted, so we crashed early. Kale offered his bed. He seemed a little uncomfortable and somewhat protective of us that night as I noticed how he rarely left our presence, which was definitely not his normal behavior. He mentioned earlier that the owners of the home were very secretive people. They made no attempt to get to know us. In the morning, he made coffee and sent us on our way.

Two days later, we arrived in Phoenix in August. It was fuckin hot—120? The water from the pool sizzled when you splashed it on the sidewalks. I had no trouble finding an electrician job as they were in high demand. Some even offered to help move me there. I told them I'd get back to them.

Kacey found an advertisement for a waitress job at a strip club. This was the first time we ever had a serious conversation about returning to that kind of work. I said, "Do you even remember how that turned out last time?"

Defensively, she replied, "This is just a waitress job. They make damn good money at places like this."

I couldn't argue that point, but I made it perfectly clear that if she wanted to reinvolve herself in that lifestyle, she would do so without Thomas and me in her life. (We were only on our honeymoon, and I'd already made threats. My insecurities were still very apparent.) Fortunately, Kacey didn't argue long. The heat was unbearable, and all I could think about was returning home.

After about a week, we returned and got back to our lives. I started a job as an electrician for a local contractor doing more residential than commercial work. Not a move forward, just sideways, as I was still an apprentice. Kacey returned to work at the tanning salon and enrolled in college again. Within a couple months, she began to have trouble at work. There were problems with the bookwork, and money was missing. I didn't know any other details as I was regrettably dismissive toward her personal troubles.

Kacey and I began to drift apart mentally. We managed to make family get-togethers but were not like we once were. I again began to be kept even further in the dark about her personal life.

Kacey began school again. Not knowing whether she quit or was fired from her job, she also began to work part-time at a bar/restaurant as a waitress. We continued to fight, but we both agreed to get counseling. Within a couple of weeks, she convinced me to move out while we sorted things out. I reluctantly moved in with a friend, our child's godfather. The honeymoon was definitely over.

> You take my words, you make them yours, then
> you twist them saying they are mine.
>
> I ask you for a reason and you refuse, and the
> truth gets lost in the nick of time.

Still unaware of the weight of the issues, I tried to make the best of it. In counseling, I sat and stared while Kacey rattled off all my wrongdoings in the past year. I rarely got a word in. It was like I was watching a tennis match. My eyes went from Kacey to the counselor, Rhonda. When I did attempt to defend myself or comment, the counselor signaled me to wait and listen. Everything I attempted to say got turned around or shut down completely. It was frustrating. I likely made the assumption most couples make while deciding to get counseling: "I'll prove I'm right. A professional will take my side." It never works that way. And it's not a contest.

(They love it when you talk. That's what you're there for. Cynically, I think, *Wow, that's easy money. Eighty bucks an hour to listen to someone.* Being broke, we only paid twenty. But I would learn that in order to get to the heart of the matter, you first have to get things off your chest. And while you do so, the counselor is listening, analyzing, and running past experiences through their head on just what might be the real issue. At least, that is what I hope they are doing. They're also establishing trust.)

Only one more session of counseling before Kacey stopped coming. I would come to find that Kacey made the recommendation, but on Rhonda's advice, we would continue with counseling on our own. I argued this, but I lost. I pleaded with Kacey to let me move back in as I tried to convince her that I was taking this seriously. She responded, "You just can't ignore a plant for a year, then dump a gallon of water on it and expect it to grow." Kacey was very perceptive.

I seemed free to come and go at our apartment and was still under the false impression that things would be fine. Kacey brought me groceries on occasion, and we had a date night once a week. We also spent time together with Thomas, often taking him to the park. I was patient. All I asked of her was that she would continue making her appointments with Rhonda. I was.

My suspicions of infidelity would become genuine when I watched our son at our apartment while she was at work. She either returned drunk and late or didn't come home at all. She told me she was staying with our friend Amanda. Amanda complied. I began to investigate her whereabouts, and her stories were not adding up, although there would be no admittance of any wrongdoing over the next few weeks.

Kacey's sister was now in town for the weekend and watching Thomas. Kacey took me out for our date night to a local restaurant. We were using a gift certificate received as one of our wedding gifts. In this heavily occupied restaurant, while waiting for our food, Kacey informed me that she was not in love with me anymore and was beginning to see someone else. She swore she had been faithful up to this point but thought we needed to separate and see other people. She was indifferent and unapologetic. I shouldn't be, but I was in shock. A normal, healthy adult should've seen this coming, but not me. As with any tragedy, I would begin my denial.

Informing me she had to meet someone and using my bewilderment to her benefit, she dropped me off at our apartment. Thomas was now sleeping. Kacey's sister asked where Kacey was. I replied, "She told me she's out deciding if she wants to be married or not." It was what I was told.

She would return that night. And as if the new guy had just turned her down (if that was possible), she told me that we were fine, that she made a mistake, that we'd get through this, and that things would get better.

This didn't appease me. I threw myself in the lion's den. I basically forced my way back into our apartment and found her life falling apart. I found paperwork with unpaid bills and credit cards, many in my name. I found warnings from college informing her that she was likely to be dropped for poor attendance and grades.

I bombarded her with questions. She ran. I interrogated our friend Amanda. All questions led up to one: "Did she cheat on me?" She disclosed to me that about a month ago, on the night of her birthday, she left the bar with a guy.

Over the next several days, with Kacey now only returning to the apartment while I was at work, I learned more of her undertakings. I was finally able to confront Kacey. We sat. I had trouble composing myself. I was in fear of her answer. I asked her, "Have you been seeing someone else?"

"No," she replied.

"Have you slept around on me?"

"No."

"What if I told you that I know for a fact you have?"

"Why? Who told you?"

"You did ... just now." Wanting it to sting, I continued, "Do you know what this means? I'm taking Thomas."

I was not a professional interrogator; Kacey was likely trying to tell me. It almost hurts worse when they don't even try to deny it. But this had to happen; no one deserved to be treated this way.

Her reaction was expected, like she suddenly had somewhere to be. She headed to the door. With her hand on the door and an evil look in her eye, she turned around to say, "Don't fight me, John. You know I'll win. I can outlast you!"

I took her words to heart and hired a lawyer.

This was not what I wanted. I had zero confidence in raising Thomas by myself. I assumed she would fight me, and I would lose. I don't think I've ever won any argument with her.

> The devil is not the doer of deeds.
> Hell is the want; Hell always needs.
> The theft of a heart is her cruelest act.
> The love she will take, and never give back.
> Run like the wind! Deny her the chance!
> Pray from a distance for you sin with a glance.
> You are not above the desires of man.
> Sin with the touch, cut off the hand.

I would become better friends with Amanda. Due to her recent squealing on her friend, Amanda was now on Kacey's shit list. But Kacey still left Thomas with her often. I pried, yet I was afraid of more truth. I found out that Kacey basically had a separate life from the one she had with me. Upon further investigation, I realized that many of these other nights that were in question, she was likely with someone else.

I was truly in hell. The bright future world that I once believed in had become a darkened pit of liars and fools, and I was the blind, naive sucker in the spotlight. I had practiced self-ridicule and loathing before, but now others could see me and pass judgment, and they were right. I couldn't even hate her because objectively, I could see that I likely had some of this coming. How vivid your recent past becomes by such a wake-up call. Momentarily, it seemed more tragic than death. It was the death of a life I envisioned. The difference is, at least death is final.

I made several more attempts to talk to Kacey. She would elude any further conversations. I wanted to at least, verbally unload my anger so she could see and hear how much this had hurt me— to have my pain validated. But she ran. I would never get to tell her. I not only had to take it, I had to keep it— by far the most selfish and harmful thing she has ever done to me.

"Tattooed all I see, all that I am, all I'll ever be…" (Pearl Jam's '*Black*' is played often.)

CHAPTER 11

Divorce

Seattle wins the Super Bowl, quite handily! I won ten bucks. Writing is very difficult. I can feel my self-esteem slipping upon every sentence. I have little definition for my passive behavior; other than my childhood did not prepare me to deal with such issues as I'm writing about. I was taught to take people at their word. Oh well, still sober, although I am still so sensitive to substance that an Advil pm can cause a slight morning hangover. Jog a mile, smoke a pack. I'm a walking satire.

—February 3, 2014,
daily journal (unedited)

I had Thomas most of the time now and spent much of my free time at the Taylor's. Through conversations with Kale's sister, Tanya (she had just been through a divorce and a cheating husband), I came to the conclusion that I had to get divorced. Although subject to interpretation, Tanya told me that even the Bible would excuse divorce due to adultery.

I filed for divorce on the grounds of adultery and mental cruelty. (Back in the '90s, I guess you still had to have a reason. It would have just been an annulment, but since a child was involved, my lawyer recommended divorce.) My lawyer also recommended that I kept track of all current interactions with Kacey and, yes, any of the dirt necessary in case she decided to fight for custody. This could get ugly. And so my journal began.

Kacey and I now both had lawyers, but nothing had been written or agreed upon. We interacted only when exchanging Thomas. I couldn't get her to pause for any conversation. I was searching for some reason for her recent behavior. Broken hearts age you quickly, and I began to analyze her not as a pissed-off soon-to-be ex-husband, but more like a parent would.

I began to reflect on our former conversations, noticing how Kacey spoke very quickly and often changed subjects before they even began. I realized she was not in the mood to be talking to me now that I'd threatened to take her son, but I was becoming aware of how her personality had recently truly changed before my eyes. If I reminded her of this, she would tell me that I didn't even know her because I never paid attention. She could be right. But I also saw how disconnected she had become from our son. When she was supposed to have him, she would leave him at the day care or with Amanda. There was more going on than two people breaking up.

Amanda had been witness to Kacey's behavior. She decided to come clean about herself and her own illness. She told me that she herself was currently on medication for bipolar disorder, or manic depression. She had reason to believe Kacey may have the same problem. She had seen more of Kacey in the past couple of months than I had. I think I had finally found something to hate.

Immediately, I began to study mental illnesses.

> Bipolar disorder, also known as bipolar affective disorder, is a mental disorder characterized by periods of elevated mood and periods of depression. The elevated mood is significant and is known as mania or hypomania depending on the severity or whether there is psychosis. During mania an individual feels or acts abnormally happy, energetic, or irritable. They often make poor thought out decisions with little regard to the consequences. The need for sleep is usually reduced. During periods of depression there may

be crying, poor eye contact with others, and a negative outlook on life. The risk of suicide among those with the disorder is high at greater than 6% over 20 years, while self-harm occurs in 30–40%. Other mental health issues such as anxiety disorder and drug misuse are commonly associated. (Wikipedia)

Ground Zero

I took over our apartment as Kacey was basically gone. Since I'd mentioned this newfound information to her of what could possibly be going on, she refused to be in my presence. Kacey usually kept things neat and clean, but the apartment was an unusual mess. There were empty cans of tuna on the floor in the kitchen, which she used to feed the cat, who also looked a little frazzled (I gave her to my parents). The cupboards were basically empty, and dirty clothes were strewn about. During one of our short conversations, I told her that I had to watch Thomas at this apartment because all his things were here and I was essentially homeless. Kacey was too busy to argue my point and basically vacated while I was at work.

I didn't grieve; I studied. This was likely a huge mistake, but I was a man. I fixed things. It was as if I couldn't get my car running and now I was digging through the manuals. I immersed myself in every available book about mental illness. Up to this point, I have had zero prior knowledge of mental illnesses other than what was displayed in movies and on the news. Currently, bipolar depression is still quite unfamiliar territory outside of psychiatry's world. I read all I could on the subject—*The Broken Brain, A Brilliant Madness, An Unquiet Mind*, to name a few. I became somewhat of a storybook psychologist.

I continued with counseling and inquired more about the subject. Rhonda, the counselor, had patience with me. I was asking more questions about Kacey and manic depression as opposed to working on myself. Rhonda understood my desperation in trying to help my wife, but she emphasized the point that she was not here—that she was not in this room. She wanted me to help myself. She was obviously trying to tell me to move on without her, but I couldn't see this at the moment. I was unconsciously choosing to help my son's mother. *I know I've never had this much use for myself.* She introduced the term *codependency*. Having already read about this, I understood it to give some reason to why I chose the company that I kept. But it was not a thing. It was a word used to describe many things. And I was not pleased with their description on how it came to be. It referred to being mistreated as a child and usually referred to being the child of an alcoholic. I quickly tried to disregard her opinion.

I read *Codependency: Adult Child of an Alcoholic.* Even the title was disconcerting. My parents were not alcoholics. I don't think my father's parents were either. My mother was adopted by her aunt, her real mother's sister. I knew nothing about that part of my mother's history and didn't really care to. I knew little to nothing about where this was supposed to take me. I believed my counselor, Rhonda, wanted me to find fault in my family's past. I likely shouldn't, but I refused. Upon discovering that I possibly had an overly passive father and a neglectful mother might explain how I came to be who I was, but I was not one to open up Pandora's box and analyze my childhood when I could only imagine how much my parents both likely improved upon my life from the way in which they were raised.

My counseling was still under Kacey's welfare payment plan, which she somehow orchestrated since before the time we were married. It was soon to run out, so I was ordered to pay over eighty dollars per hour in order to continue. I made ten dollars per hour. It wasn't going to happen.

I was wide open to any other suggestions. I rarely slept. I'd lost whatever weight that wasn't necessary for my survival. I indulged in caffeine and cigarettes. I neurotically searched the self-help section at the library on occasion, absorbing anything and everything from codependency to mental illnesses and manic depression, all while experiencing true single parenting. Kacey had already begun to withdraw from her time with him. Thomas was now only fifteen months old. We were married less than three months ago.

My infrequent conversations with Kacey now mostly concerned Thomas as she told me when she was going to see him (we still hadn't been to court). It was two o'clock on a Tuesday. Earlier, she informed me she was picking him up from day care. I was in between service calls in my work truck. Through learning more about this illness, I was becoming cautious of her actions concerning Thomas. No, I was extremely paranoid! I was worried she'd run off with him. Not having a plan if she did, I hid my truck out of view from the day care. Yeah, I was a stalking her, but I believed I was justified. Kacey and her new guy pulled up. Kacey got out wearing a bright-colored skirt, orange or pink, something she would never wear. Her hair was curling-iron curled, and she was wearing heels and carrying a purse. She had bright-red lipstick on. Yeah, gorgeous, but I barely recognized her. I'd never seen her look like this in the time I knew her. I wrote down the license plates and made a mental picture of the truck. Confused, I spent the afternoon worrying, but Thomas was thankfully at day care when I arrived at five thirty.

A couple of days later, I would see this same truck across an intersection while waiting at a red light. She was with her new man. She gave me a look that I'll never forget. She had a gleam in her eye and an arrogant smile that said "I told you so. Now start your suffering." Oh, I would!

I thought to myself, *Who the hell is she?* I claimed I knew her well. Her favorite color was orange, not for clothes, just the color. Her favorite song was *Fast Car* by Tracy Chapman. She loved dolphins. She laughed loud like Julia Roberts. She loved intimacy during the rain. She also used to hate what infidelity did to families and relationships. But whatever hatred that may have existed inside her was now directed entirely toward me.

I was her brand-new number 1 enemy. I was now the guy trying to take her son while sitting in judgment of her behavior like I was some overbearing parent. And if she was in a manic state of mind, relative to cocaine high, I was the guy trying to remove that feeling. For that reason alone, which didn't occur to me at the time, I could now understand her anger. I was not yet beginning to forgive her; I was beginning to understand her.

I would convince Kacey to meet me at a small, right off campus bar. I didn't know the reason why we were here; I guess we were discussing Thomas and our future apart. With my newfound knowledge, I was truly analyzing her behavior now. I wanted to witness this thing called manic depression.

I somehow managed to keep her talking, mostly subjects that only needed simple answers. She gave me a couple of phone numbers as to where she could be reached in case of an emergency. This was a difficult situation. I wanted to unload my anger, but if I were to bring up anything serious, she was bound to run. I felt I was making progress toward a real conversation, one that just might convince her to see herself needing help.

There was a young girl, maybe nine years old, who began striving to get Kacey's attention. (Didn't she know how important our conversation was? I've been struggling to be heard and understood by others since this happened. Don't interrupt me. This is how the world conspires against me!) Kacey easily accepted this young girl's thirst for attention as she likely feared my impending words. Kacey was eager for a distraction. This began a routine between the two of them that would completely remove any serious discussion from taking place. Their interaction continued long enough that even the parents of the young girl were taking notice and becoming uncomfortable. This was not even close to Kacey's normal behavior.

I returned home confused and disappointed. I guess I was hoping to see something in Kacey's eyes. Hoping that if she could focus on me long enough, she'd recognize me as the guy she agreed to marry less than three months ago. She struggled to make eye contact with me. For the one second we did make eye contact, I saw nothing but distance, like she was just drunk. I didn't see manic depression, as if you could. I didn't see love. I didn't see hate. I only saw indifference. The Kacey I knew was just not there.

Beginning to truly believe in manic depression, I again consulted Amanda. I asked her what could be done in Kacey's case. From her experience, she said that if she was currently in a manic state, there wasn't much I could do other than hospitalization.

Days later, and I honestly don't know how we managed it, but before Kacey knew what was happening, we were all in my Blazer on our way to see Amanda's doctor. Kacey was livid. If it was a four-door truck, she would've bailed. She'd never been physically afraid of me as I had recently become like a punching bag to her. She was letting me have it verbally, but her usual brilliant depiction of what an ass I was, was even somewhat distorted and confusing. Her voice was hoarse and worn-out. Her sentences tended to run on top of one another, and her biggest complaint was that she was scheduled to go snow skiing somewhere this weekend with her boyfriend. She believed she's just angry, and there was truly no way of knowing the difference. We'd basically abducted her. I was told by Amanda to keep my mouth shut and just drive.

Somehow, Amanda managed to convince Kacey to check herself in just for the night. We legally had no right to force her to go. She made no mention of causing harm to herself or others, unless Amanda lied to the staff. Kacey would even put my name down as a contact.

I have no idea why she went along with us. Even now I wonder if she was just trying to get us to stop helping her by proving us wrong. Maybe everything was happening too fast, and part of her felt somewhat afraid for herself. Then there was the slight chance that she had no idea what was going on at that time. It's all my speculation. She was given medication and would release herself against the doctor's recommendation the next morning.

Days later, Amanda would give me a composition she had come across while she, herself, was hospitalized for manic depression. It is an insightful depiction of a life I too can relate to.

It was titled "Please Hear What I'm Not Saying."

> Don't be fooled by me. Don't be fooled by the thousand masks, masks that I'm afraid to take off and none of them is me. Pretending is an art that's second nature with me, but don't be fooled, for God's sake don't be fooled. I give you the impression that I am secure, that all is sunny and unruffled with me, within as well as without.

Confidence is my name and coolness is my game; that the waters calm and I am in command and that I need no one. But don't believe me. Please.

My surface may seem smooth, but my surface is my mask. Beneath this lies no compliance. Beneath dwells the real me in confusion, in fear, and in aloneness. But I hide this. I don't want anyone to know it. I panic at the thought of my weakness and fear of being exposed. That is why I frantically create a mask to hide behind, a nonchalant, sophisticated façade to help me pretend, to shield me from the glance that knows. But such a glance is precisely my salvation, my only salvation. And I know it. That is if it's followed by acceptance, it is followed by love. It's the only thing that will assure me of what I can't assure myself; that I am worth something.

But I don't tell you this. I don't dare. I am afraid to. I am afraid your glance will not be followed by acceptance and love. I'm afraid you'll think less of me. That you'll laugh at me. And your laugh would kill me. I'm afraid that deep down I am nothing, that I am no good, and that you will see this and reject me. So I play my game, my desperate game, with a façade of assurance without and a trembling child within. And so begins the parade of masks. And my life becomes a front.

I idly chatter to you in the suave tone of surface talk. I tell you everything that is really nothing and nothing of what's everything, of what's crying within me; so when I'm going through my routine, do not be fooled by what I am saying. Please listen carefully and try to hear what I am not saying, what I'd like to be able to say, for what survival I need to say, but I can't say.

I dislike hiding. Honestly! I dislike the superficial game I'm playing, the phony game. I'd really like to be genuine and spontaneous, and me, but you've got to hold out your hand, even though that is the last thing I seem to want. Only you can wipe away from my eyes the blank stare of breathing death. Only you can call me into aliveness. Each time you're kind and gentle and encouraging, each time you try to understand, because you really care, my heart begins to grow wings, very small wings, very feeble wings, but wings. With your sensitivity and sympathy, and your power of understanding, you can breathe life into me. I want you to know that.

I want you to know how important you are to me, how you can be the creator of the person that is me if you choose to. Please choose to. You alone can break down the walls behind which I tremble. You alone can remove my mask. You alone can release me from my shadow world of panic, and insecurities and uncertainty, from my lonely person. Don't pass me by. Please don't pass me by.

It will not be easy for you. A long conviction of worthlessness builds strong walls. The nearer you approach me, the blinder I strike back. I fight against the very thing I cry out for. But I am told that love is stronger than walls, and in this lies my hope. Please try to beatdown those walls with firm hands, but with gentle hands for a child is very sensitive. Who am I? You may wonder. I am someone you know very well. For I am every man you meet and I am every woman you meet. (unknown author)

Later, I would read this to Kale. He told me that it sounded like me. And he was right. But if it was written by someone with manic depression, I seemed to have missed out on the excitement of mania.

I should not have read this. This was written by someone who wanted help, someone who was at rock bottom, someone who possibly regretted or at least admitted to feeling different. Because of this composition, I saw this person that I believe existed inside Kacey, even though I might be wrong.

I would try to read this composition to Kacey, but she would run. I would like to think, at this time, that I was driven by a desire to help someone, to reconnect a child and his mother, to do the right thing. Somewhere in my mind, I believed that Kacey needed to recognize what she was doing as a huge mistake so I alone would not have to be responsible for my son. I was not up for that. I was very afraid. I had this secret belief that when she was well, she was still the better parent. If she could get better, maybe I won't have to. Because I didn't know what was wrong with me, if anything. I understood I was heartbroken, but I believed I was still logical. This recent information I'd acquired about manic depression, they made it sound fairly easy to become a normal, healthy person again. And it had become obvious at this point; we were both too young, too crazy to be good parents. What the hell did I know about parenting? Personally, I would feel much more comfortable being the weekend father who paid the bills. I had never taken care of anyone, including myself. But I refused to release my son to anyone who was not willing to fight for him.

In Kacey's eyes, I fell right into the category of a man who couldn't let her go, an insecure, weak man who refused to accept that it was over. She likely witnessed this behavior before, not just from me, but from former boyfriends. And I couldn't win that argument if I tried. I understand it now, but at this point in time, I truly didn't know the difference.

CHAPTER 12

Wisdom

I tried my best to give it some space and tried to get back to who I was. I called Kale. I understood he was home for the week. We hadn't seen much of each other but spoke on the phone, so he was up to date on my current situation. I had confided in him throughout my relationship with Kacey. He knew how much I cared for her; all the while, I was still trying to maintain my image as a strong, confident man. He gave advice as he also had problems of his own with his ex and their son. Although I spoke ill of Kacey at times to him, I couldn't get him to. He'd never been like that. He did understand compassion, but it was in his own way.

Kale answers the phone, "Yeah?"

"Hey, let's do something tonight," I command.

"All right ... You gonna bitch about your ex–ole lady all night?" He is direct, but funny.

"I might for a while. Why? Is that a problem?"

"For how long?" he asks.

I reply, "How about an hour?"

"All right. You get one hour. But that's it!"

It was Halloween. Thomas was with my parents. My brother was running the karaoke in town. The first drink was free if you were in costume. We didn't plan ahead to dress up as anything, so Kale dug through his trunk in the parking lot outside the bar. Shuffling through his work clothes, he found a hard hat, gloves, safety glasses, and a hi-vis vest.

"Here, put this stuff on. You'll look like a real electrician, a lineman."

I put it all on and say, "Shit, I look like one of the village people."

"What's wrong with that?" he asks.

"I can't wear this. I look like the gay one."

Laughing, he replies, "I thought they were all gay. Ah, you look like a lineman."

"What are you gonna wear?" I ask.

"Nothin'. I got money."

We would end this night with some much-needed 2:00 a.m. gravel-road philosophy. It seemed we had even more in common now that we'd both had a 'she-devil' suck the life force out of us. Kale told me that his ex-girlfriend also mentioned to him that she had also once been diagnosed as bi-polar. We compared notes. Without considering his own dilemma, I asked him how it was possible for a mother to walk away from her own kid. He thought about it. "Maybe they think it's better that way."

"But it's not," I replied.

"Maybe it is, maybe it isn't, but if that's how they think, there's nothing you can do about it."

He was tiring from my questions. We started a religious conversation. Due to my unanswered prayers and my frustration in convincing others to understand my situation, I told Kale that if I held the power of God, if I could magically freeze everyone who came into contact with Kacey and quickly inform them of how a boy was missing his mother due to this medical condition called manic depression, and if they just took a minute to help, to not treat Kacey as if nothing was wrong, to help point her toward medical help, then they would reunite this innocent boy with his mother. If they knew this, they would help.

Kale replied, "Yeah, good luck with that!"

Because in my mind, I thought if I could get the world to stop and believe that I knew something others didn't, I could change the world. Further into this heavy conversation, I turned again to Kale, and while physically acting it out, I asked him, "What do you suppose would happen if I literally rose up above a crowd and said, 'God is speaking through me. Stop your hatred and judgment. I am proof of him. I am floating above you through God's will'?"

Kale quickly responds in his sly tone, "They'd shoot ya right outta the sky!"

We shared a laugh.

The Black Crowes played on the radio. Kale cranked it up. I told him that this band didn't impress me. "C'mon, man!" He sang along, "She'll tell you she's an orphan, after you meet her family. She talks to angels... You can't relate to that?" I would quickly learn to appreciate their music. The next song was a form of rap/rock music. I sarcastically asked, "And what's the meaning of this song?"

He began bobbing his head. "This song says, 'Fuck it! Quit thinkin' 'bout shit and bang your head!'" Ah... true wisdom. I enjoyed the break.

At home, I began receiving bills in the mail for things I'd never purchased—Dayton's, Limited, Victoria Secrets. I recently found several cards around the apartment in my name and a forged signature. I inquired about the purchases with the retailers and was told since they were in my name, I was responsible. (I know. It is bullshit. Forgery is still forgery. At the time, I was sure they were just hoping I'd pay up. And yeah, I know what you're thinking, and you're right: the Victoria Secrets card hurt me the most.)

I was broke. The total was around $1,500.

I mentioned this to my lawyer. He told me to contact the police to see if there was anything they could do. At the cop shop, I was informed that even though it was obviously not my signature, there was not much that could be done. I would likely have to take Kacey to court. An officer went on to tell me he was currently investigating a case that involved my address. He asked me if I thought Kacey was capable of stealing the identity of the prior tenant from our apartment. I told him, at this point, anything was possible. I was told to contact him if I learned any new information.

I would receive a phone call from Dr. Benet. He was the attending doctor when Kacey was brought in. He was also Amanda's doctor. He asked how Kacey was doing. He was hoping to see her again. I informed him of the last couple of weeks and told him I didn't know where she was or what she was doing. She hadn't seen her son in a while.

I asked for his professional opinion of her. "What did you find out the night we brought her in?" He first confirmed that I was listed as a contact then proceeded to give me his opinion, although he wished he had more time with her. He said she wasn't very cooperative. He found that she wasn't on drugs and said it was most likely that she was in a manic state of manic depression. He gave her medication to get her to calm down but said she definitely needed to keep coming back in order to find the proper prescription. He would give me his personal number. I told him I'd pass that message on when and if I would see her.

I was now working alone in our local mall changing ballasts in the hallway light fixtures. Kacey recognized my run down, rusted out utility truck outside and approached out of nowhere. "Hey, you want me to be medicated, right?" she asked.

"I want you to be well," I replied.

She looked tired and disheveled, most likely medicated. "Can you loan me twenty bucks to refill my prescription?"

I responded, "Your doctor is looking for you. How do you know what you're supposed to take?"

Agitated and impatient, as if I was her last chance, while patting her pocket, she stated, "I talked to him. He said to refill this one until I see him again." She turned away. Her body language said she was leaving. She started off, "Fine. You're the one that wants me on this shit."

"Hold on." I was truly hoping we would get to have a longer discussion. I didn't even have time to discuss the credit card issues. I reluctantly dug for a twenty.

Handing her the money, looking her directly in the eyes, I politely but sincerely said, "I'm glad you're trying."

She swiped the twenty from my hand. "Whatever." She left as quickly as she walked in. (Hootie and the Blowfish's "Let Her Cry" played on the radio in the background.)

I shared the details of my credit card issues with Amanda. She watched Thomas regularly and came and went freely to and from my apartment. I gave her the latest information about these credit cards and told her that the cops were looking into security videos at an electronics store, trying to see who stole the prior tenant's identity. Apparently, whoever did this bought items there and returned them for cash. I also asked if she could watch Thomas on Wednesday nights while I played city league basketball. Surprisingly, she now told me that she was busy but referred me to her own current babysitter. I would grow somewhat suspicious of Amanda.

This new babysitter agreed to watch Thomas. She was a senior in high school, and after a few conversations, she disclosed that her mother also suffered from manic depression. It turned out we even shared the same counselor—small, crazy world.

(We're not all just crazy, by the way. Going in to see the shrink is like being a tourist on the road—if you sense something wrong with your vehicle and happen to stop and see a mechanic, they're bound to find something; it's their job. And I haven't met anyone who can't use a tune-up now and again. It just seemed that since my recently acquired information, I tended to initiate conversations in which everyone I knew had a relative or friend with some type of relatable psychological issue. I had yet to meet anyone who was free of this. I was astonished by the magnitude of mental illnesses and disturbed by how secretive it was kept. How were we to remedy anything if it was taboo to discuss? My new sitter also gave me insight relating to what a teenager went through living with mental illness in the family. She would eventually introduce me to her friend and classmate Laura, who would also help share the babysitting workload. Laura and I would become close. Through her admiration of my writings and poetry, she would have me believe that I was, at least, a poet. Laura would eventually become my muse—next book.)

Three-Eighths Hole

In November of '94, around Thanksgiving week, Kale, Amanda, and I met up at Rob's bar. Thomas was with my parents. Kacey's whereabouts were unknown. I only had her work number. She was likely living with her new boyfriend in the city, but still with me in my mind. I saw Kale once on Halloween, and now he was back from Colorado. His next job was to be in California. He brought an ample supply of weed with him, more than I'd ever seen him possess. I'd never known him to sell weed, but he was likely looking to supply some of our friends whom we'd mooched from often. He had never really been involved in distributing weed at this level, not to my knowledge anyway. He'd now been driving for twelve hours and was noticeably tired and weary from the road. I had always questioned his driving ability and tonight it was visibly clear how tired he was. But I only asked once for him to ride with us and stay in my parents' basement. Before we left Rob's, Kale hesitated before deciding. "Ah, I've already put in twelve hours on the road today. What's another half hour?" he said.

We parted ways.

At about 4:00 a.m., my parents' phone rang. My mother woke me to tell me Kale was on the phone.

"It's four a.m. What the hell you doin'?" I asked.

"I passed out and hit an approach with my truck. Fucked it up bad!"

"Are you okay?"

"No. I think I broke my ankle, and I got like a three-eighths hole in my head!"

"What?!"

"Yeah, I can stick my pinkie in it and poke my skull. I need you to drive out there and make sure I didn't leave any trace of weed behind."

"Where's the truck? How the hell did you make it home?"

"It's about three or four miles away from here. I couldn't get my feet to cooperate with me, so I had to walk sideways all the way home. You gotta get out there and check my truck!"

"I'm not goin' out there now. I'm still drunk!" I replied.

"Send Amanda out there! She was sober, right?"

I handed Amanda the phone. Kale informed her of the truck's whereabouts. I stayed home with Thomas. She tried to find the truck, but not having been familiar with the area, she had no luck.

Early the next morning, we made the trip to Joan's to see Kale. He was in bad shape. I insisted on taking him to the hospital. He was hesitant as he feared the law would find him there. He was more stubborn and paranoid than he'd ever been. Knowing he was in no shape to kick my ass, I got aggressive with him.

"Look, you dumbfuck! You can't even walk! Your ankles are broken. There is no other option!" I basically had to carry him to my Blazer.

He didn't want to go anywhere near the truck now as he feared repercussions from the law. We found another friend to hold the majority of his weed for him while we went to the hospital. I was right: two broken ankles and several stitches.

They would keep him for two days. When we picked him up, he did not want to return home. He was still unusually cautious of the law and asked if he could stay with me in my parents' basement. I made arrangements with my mother as I was going back to college town with Thomas on Monday. I explained to my mother that he was worried about getting in trouble for not reporting the accident. The cops had to be looking for him, and Kale thought this was the safest place. My mother hadn't been a fan of our local law enforcement since my trial a few years ago, so she and my father agreed to keep tabs on Kale for a couple of weeks.

I returned on the weekend, and Kale was fortunately moving around on crutches quite well for wearing two casts on his legs. On the second weekend, he left money for groceries with my mother and sincerely thanked her for her hospitality. The truck was apparently hauled to his mother's home by a friend over a week ago. He would spend the rest of his healing time there.

I would learn that Kacey moved in with her boyfriend in the city about an hour away. We were to appear in court a couple of times, but she failed to respond to requests from my lawyer. I informed my lawyer about my fears of Kacey's possible illness and recent behavior, so on his advice, I had my divorce decree written with me having primary physical custody of Thomas. Kacey was to have secondary custody with weekend and summer visitation based solely on the condition that she received counseling and continued to counsel until her doctor would recommend that she was fit to have longer, unsupervised visits. He again recommended that I keep a record of interactions and phone conversations with Kacey in case she would decide to fight for custody.

Kacey hadn't been seen or heard from in a few weeks. I would hear about sightings in bars through friends, yet she hadn't made any serious attempts to contact me or to argue over custody or see our son. This was not like her.

She would miss our confirmed court date. Through my persistent outreaching by phone, she agreed to meet at my lawyer's office. She eventually signed the necessary paperwork without argument.

As we walked out of the office, sarcastically, Kacey asked, "Happy now?"

I replied, "What? Did you expect me not to divorce you?"

She solemnly looked at the ground. "No."

I went on, "Look, whatever you think should've happened, you gotta 'get right'. Thomas is only a year and half old. He's not gonna know any of this, but I'm gonna need your help. I don't know what the fuck I'm doin' either. Get your shit together so you can help me."

"Yeah, yeah," she replied while walking away.

My lawyer informed me that there was nothing written saying she couldn't still fight for custody in the future. He knew me well, so he reminded me to be on my best behavior. We would have until January 15 to change our minds about the details of custody and divorce. She was also ordered to pay one hundred dollars per month for child support.

I would spend Christmas at my parents' home in my hometown, and much of all the family were there. Upon arrival, while removing my one-and-a-half-year-old son's jacket, Thomas began to notice all the familiar faces. He began to look at my sister, my sister-in-law, and my mother, all individually, quickly turning his head. He started to cry profusely. I felt my stomach turn. I couldn't do anything for him. My sister-in-law finally walked out with him. I had to leave the room. It was a moment I wouldn't forget. It is why I've been trying so hard; not to have his mother here for Christmas but at least, for him to know she was somewhere waiting for him. If I was to ever hate her, I did at this moment.

I read the composition "Please Hear What I'm Not Saying" to my family. I guess I wanted to inform them about mental illnesses. And I truly didn't want them hating Kacey. Also being cautious and somewhat paranoid, I would warn my parents about Kacey. It was a 'be-here-now' moment. I told them that I didn't trust her and that no matter what Kacey would say or do, if she were to show up here, they were not to leave Thomas alone with her. I knew my father would show certain weakness in such a situation. I made them both look me in the eyes and promise. My limited knowledge of manic depression put me in fear of the idea that she might take him away and never look back. She was well versed in getting lost and had no trouble finding an accomplice. And my imagination was always more dramatic than the truth. Hope for the best; plan for the worst.

CHAPTER 13

Journal Break

"Like a cloud dropping rain, I'm discarding all thoughts. I'll dry up, leaving puddles on the ground."

—Pearl Jam

The sickness has returned in full force. It's Saturday. Wednesday, I began to lose faith in everything written. My ability to create completely disappeared as did my memories. I can't tell when it comes, I can only tell when it leaves. I exercised yesterday afternoon, rode the dirt bike, ate the same food, didn't drink, and yet I couldn't feel anything. It is so powerful that even the perfect weather goes unrecognized. Physical ailments are apparent; body aches, slight head ache, tired, but can't actually sleep. Even food loses its flavor. How in the fuck is that possible? You can't read, you certainly can't write. It takes all you can do to sit and watch TV in which you will gain nothing and remember nothing. You are truly just buying time until it's over.

Last night, I started to feel normal after eating dinner and watching a movie. When I start to feel good, only then do I recognize that I was feeling bad. After years of this consistent depression, you'd think I would find a way to make it disappear by changing my environment, my company, my food intake, my sleep, but nothing keeps it at bay and nothing makes it leave. It seems to have a life of its own and it is merciless. This morning it's sunny and 70 degrees. Birds are chirping, the gophers are frolicking, life is continuing with or without my involvement.

I feel it fleeing me now as I write this but it seems it has nothing to do with what I do or how I think. I can't be responsible for its presence because that would also make me feel inadequate for my inability to make it leave.

The closest psychological definition I've ever heard: Anxiety disorder accompanied with depression. I have nothing to be anxious about. I'm single, my son is home and doing fine, sun is abundant, there is plenty of food in the fridge and I am not in need of anything; yet I am sick. If I was working my normal job as an electrician somewhere, these last few days would be when I start to hate everything about my job. My mind then reaches out to find the source of depression. Is it my asshole boss, my coworkers, my parenting skills, my overall choice in careers? I used to think the anxiety began from internalizing my thoughts at work—by withholding true thoughts and opinions about the job and my coworkers during the controversial decisions one has to make while on the job. Therefore, I would assume anxiety is causing my depression. This is when I would take a day or two off from work and stare at the TV trying to let it take its course. I have no explanation to give the boss when I return and I can't ask for time off ahead of time because I never know when it's coming. All of this has repercussions and truly affects my life. If I were with a woman, she would likely tire of this behavior in time and leave. This has been proven. I have begged for its mercy, I have prayed, I have fasted, and I have taken medication. It is larger than life. Depression does not need anxiety to exist. But worst of all it does, right now, it is constantly trying to stop me from writing.

Yes, I've been on medication. In 2010, I was taking citalopram for over a year. I dated again. I acquired and maintained several relationships with some lasting up to about 3 months, which seems to be enough time to figure out if it the relationship was going to work. My job became easier. I drank a lot less. I felt quite normal. No complaints other than my meds definitely affected my sex drive. It also kept me from reconnecting with my past while trying to write. Obsessive thoughts can be beneficial for writing, but my creative ability was absent. Ironically, the part of the brain that may give you a specific ability is also the part that thinks 'you suck.' I didn't hear the 'you suck' part for many months, but I seem to need it to write. So here I am.

I have an urge to go for a ride on Shine (Harley), and hit the bar on the way back; very sick of myself right now. The motorcycle has a way of forcing you to only think ahead. There is no chance of reflecting on self- ridicule while in traffic on Shine or climbing hills with the Honda. Thoughts have to be centered on survival. Although temporary, it's definitely an escape.

People like me unconsciously seek out what it was that last made us consistently happy. This is likely the reason I pursued the company of the mother of my child. Whether she was with me or not, I would seek out her words and her attention in order to feel somewhat normal; to distract me from myself. Even if she actively hated me, it would draw my attention away from the way I'm feeling. I also do not want to be the only one in charge of my son. I know myself. There will be times when I have to be alone, truly alone. To hide away in a room and let the hours of sickening self- talk and ridicule subside. He's a year and half old at this time in the story. He needs constant supervision and attention.

People will conform out of nowhere to help me. People are seemingly good (Amanda), until you question their motives.

"Depression," February 8, 2014, journal entry (a couple of average weeks in my life)

Sleep?

Sleep escapes me as my mind races through the past, the future, and the never ending awareness that I am still awake. Like love, the more I pursue it, the more distant it becomes. I focus my thoughts on lighthearted events, daily routines, the humor in friends, but all is interrupted by the last few deep breathes I take before entering dreamland. Then begins the routine again....

> Well, I got that out of my system. Rode shine to the casino to buy cheap cigarettes. Stopped at a bar near my temporary home on the way back and drank tap beer until I liked myself again. Do not feel anything like depression today. I feel a slight hangover and it is nothing compared to how I felt yesterday and the day before. I feel like I can accomplish something again. Maybe not today, but the positive thoughts are coming back.

I'm okay. I will likely try medication again when this is done. (February 9, 2014)

Not quite out of it yet. Doing everything I've learned to change my perspective but I'm still in the funk. The only thing you can do when depressed is be depressed. Fuck! I'm trying to go back and edit the beginning but I can't even stand to look at it. I want to erase it all. Just might have to get medicated before continuing. Hope not. Have to go back home to work soon. Six days and I'm not better. (February 11, 2014)

Hey God?

Is this all a big joke?
Should I burn this when done?
The bitterness growing; the hatred from my son.
Did the complexity of my mind come through my parent's DNA?
Is chemical intercourse why I'm here today?
If not, let me be simple.
Let me love something easy.
Grant me peace through direction.
Or just let me be.

(This was not intended to be about me; the journey of self-discovery.)

Happy Birthday to me! Just read last journal entry. Wow! Think twice before you ask me how I feel! Easy, John. I'm fine. Been editing here and there. Can't tell if I'm 'right' just yet, tho. Got on the Advil pm for a few days. Shit is addicting. Couldn't sleep without it. Think I'm good. Was joking with Joan on the phone about me possibly having pms. Ha!! Average now is about a week every month. I'll bring that up with the doc next time.

I think it's possibly only the second time in 25 years that I haven't gotten drunk on my birthday; afraid of the hangover costing me time. Onward... (February 16, 2014)

(January 28, 2015) Hello, again! I'm finally back in AZ. Notice the date! (Year later) I've been here almost a month now, going over everything written up to this point. What's ahead of this was obviously done in a hurry so I'm choosing to begin again here.

I'm okay. I'm still somewhat of a slave to my moods but since sometime last summer, I haven't had real depression last longer than a day or two. And it's likely what normal 'healthy' people call having a bad day. I'm here again with Tobi and my bikes. No TV, only intermittent Internet on my phone. I can hardly tune in a radio station. I'm farther north than last time so the weather is only a frigid 65 for a high. I'll still drink with the locals, about once a week. I jog or ride my bicycle daily. And I'll still have a day or two in between where I can't write and nothing makes sense. But overall, I'm in a good place in my life right now. I'll survive.

I hopefully, won't interrupt this story with my personal depressing shit until the end. There is plenty of that to come. Trust that I'm okay.

They call it an anxiety disorder coupled with
   depression.
A mind trapped inside a false face, a mind far too
   obsessive.
A lifetime of worry and guilt over nothing,
Fear of embarrassment, afraid to do something.
Self-medicating, pour me some truth

Smoke myself funny and bring back my youth.
No longer stuck in the rut of overthinking a
    thought.
Acting, not thinking, learning, not taught.
The beginning has begun, I now see who I am,
Still a stranger to myself, I want to be this new
    man.

CHAPTER 14

Six Months in the Life

In January of 1995, my divorce was finally official. They make you wait sixty days. I don't know why. You can get a permit for a handgun a hell of lot quicker than a divorce. The bill for the wedding pictures just arrived. What a waste. I never did have enough money to pay back the credit cards. Some dropped their case against me, while others turned me in to the credit bureau. My credit would take a slight hit.

Kale and his brother Steve were now working in California for the same substation construction company. They were again working with our longtime friend Dan. Dan was in my sister's class and had been a friend of ours since high school. In 1983, straight out of high school, he joined this construction company when they were working nearby and had been on the road with them ever since. He has a home now in my same hometown. His dad and my dad were cousins, so I guess we are somehow related. He might laugh at this, but he had been and is still one of my more responsible close friends.

Their job often took them to distant places throughout the Midwest and southwest as far as Arizona and California. Much like Kale's former job building grain bins, they had a core of steady workers who traveled with the company. The rest were often hired locally, mostly as general laborers from the same area as the job location. These jobs always varied in length of time. I wouldn't pay much attention to how long they were gone or where they were. I only saw them when they returned home in between jobs or on holidays. Kale and Steve had both been with Dan, or at least the same company, off and on for over a year now. In January, they were all on the same job in California.

Through conversations with Kale, he had made some comments about how he thought he should be making more money than his older brother because he was an actual classified lineman who was now educated in this trade. The job required several areas of construction work as there were only a few actual linemen on the job. Kale and Steve ended up in a physical scuffle, likely over this issue, with Kale as the aggressor when they were at their mother's over Christmas. It was short-lived, however, because Joan was home at the time and likely hollered "All right!" at the appropriate time. I know this happened several times in their youth, but it had been years since they were physical with each other. It was apparent that Kale was unhappy.

It was around this time that I learned that Steve had a son on the way in Minnesota and had intentions to marry the mother. Kale was still trying to keep the peace with his son and ex-girlfriend. He had seen them on occasion but rarely discussed details about his visits with me.

Sometime during the holiday break, Kale and I ended up at the bar near his mother's. Thomas was with Joan, Tanya, and Tanya's daughter at the Taylor home. I brought Thomas there often. There was a wedding dance across the street from the bar. Kale had a new girlfriend with him. We all toked from a homemade can pipe, and it was apparently really good weed. I was temporarily lost in my surroundings. I hadn't done it in a while, and I was almost too high to enjoy being high. I didn't feel like I had in the past couple of months as that was likely all I'd been looking for.

It was fairly busy at the dance, but we were unfamiliar with the wedding parties and the crowd, so we ended up at the bar across the street. We attempted to play pool. All three of us were in the spirit world. Kale was leaning way back in his chair with a relaxed smile on his face. I was sitting across the table. A stranger walked up and leaned in to tell Kale something that I couldn't hear. He had a friend with him who wore a cast on his arm. I could make out the guy pointing at the front door and then to the back door while he was talking. I found out later he was asking Kale to either step out this door or that door to see just how bad he was. I leaned in to listen.

With his eyes half-closed and barely lifting his head, Kale slowly responds, "Look, dude. You're gonna have to hit me right where I'm sittin' ... 'cause I am fuuucked up!" This 'dude' and his friend were both well-built. They looked at me and likely noticed that my eyes couldn't even focus long enough to comprehend the situation. They continued to talk for a minute as I attempted to come back to reality. I was aware there could be trouble, but like Kale, there wasn't much I could do or wanted to risk doing. Luckily, they left us without a physical confrontation.

The next day at Joan's, recalling the night before, I asked Kale what that was all about. Showing little concern, Kale replied, "I don't know, man. I musta pissed him off."

"Why'd you decide to let it go?"

"'Cause I was a fuckin' mess! I told him where I lived and that if he was still pissed off in the morning and wanted to fuck me up, he could come and find me out here."

"Damn. I wish I would've known what was happenin'," I declared.

"Why? What were you gonna do? Ha-ha! You were like a fuckin' noodle!"

"You sure you didn't say somethin' to him? I mean, why would he want to kick your ass?" I asked.

Agitated, Kale responded, "I don't know, man. Maybe I was eyeballin' him earlier. Who gives a shit? Why you gotta know everything? Why you always gotta be 'Johnny-with-the-news'? You writin' a book or somethin'?"

After a long pause, I replied, "I might."

"Well, let it go. We're lucky we didn't get thumped!"

Although these encounters likely happened often to Kale, it still seemed unusual to me. I couldn't understand how strangers walked up to someone and provoked a fight just because they may have heard on the street that the guy was tough. It's possible that they were friends with someone Kale thumped in the past. Who knows? It would seem there are always repercussions after a fight, win or lose.

It never ends. But I've likely given this more thought than Kale ever did.

I'd always had the feeling that this wasn't how normal people should live. I didn't know then and still don't know if these bizarre encounters are worthy of belonging in a book. Whether these stories are for entertainment or for enlightenment, I knew that I wanted to remember them as I have always been intrigued by those who have no fear of differing from the norm.

In the following months, Kale and Steve would return to California, and my conversations with him were becoming infrequent. This could be due to my self-loathing. Feeling sorry for yourself is like having the flu; people will show concern, but they'd rather not be around you or hear your shit. I didn't blame Kale for not calling as often as I myself was not above it. Besides, my mind was still on Kacey.

I was still in the fog of a failed marriage, single parenting, and a broken heart. I thought I was stronger than this. I refused to accept that she was gone and that I couldn't save her from herself. I did know that she was not who she used to be. I still remembered her as the highly intelligent, beautiful girl who tried to help homeless people, rescued abandoned animals, and loved children. I still believed I was not wrong about her. She was a good person. Her son should know her.

If I had her number, I would continue to call Kacey monthly, just to see if she was counseling and hopefully, wanting to see her son. I also had yet to receive any child support. I would lure her into reconciliation with her son, and then when she was getting closer to seeing him, I'd tell her she needed to follow what was written in our divorce decree. I could hear her vindicated frustration over the phone. I was unintentionally toying with her. I pretended to know what I'm doing. I didn't have the required ability to see this from the outside—just like Kacey. And by now, the sound of my voice must be like nails on a chalkboard to her. I couldn't get her to talk about anything longer than a few seconds. In the heat of one of our short face-to-face conversations, in my frustration as she was again running away, I asked her if she planned all this just to fuck up my life.

She paused on her way out to look me in the eye as she stated, "John, you give me way more credit than I deserve!" She went on to tell me that instead of trying to save the world, I should learn more about codependency. Although I ignored her in the past, I currently took everything she said to heart.

One should never associate a mental illness with a lack of intelligence—quite the opposite. Apart from Kacey's prior college days, she'd never carried a grade point average lower than 4.0. Kale and Kacey both are two of the most intelligent people I know, insightful and perceptive, obviously not because of their lifestyle decisions, but because of their insight, how quickly they can find reason, their perception of others, and their judgment of character. When either of them would be provoked with an awkward confrontation, I would find myself smiling with anticipation. Kacey would articulate with such precision about how wrong this stranger's choice of words or actions were that she would leave them stunned and speechless. You could tell they'd never had their ass chewed by a professional. Kale chose to let the stranger carry on with his ridiculousness until slowly leaning in, looking him in the eye, and with his Clint Eastwood–like direct manner, he would say, "Are you *tryin'* to piss me off?" Because I lacked this skill, I was drawn to those who have mastered the art of confrontation. And I began to intensify my search for any reason I might lack these abilities.

> Codependency—Relationships that are a type of dysfunctional helping relationship where one person supports or enables another person's addiction, poor mental health, immaturity, irresponsibility, or under-achievement. Among the characteristics of Codependency, the most common theme is excessive reliance on the other people for approval and identity. (Wiki on codependency)

Well, Kacey was right on. Although I don't know how anyone can be excluded from such issues at some point in your life. If you're in a relationship, you tend to become reliant on the other person. It should not reach such a level as to form your identity or risk your own health. And I'm well aware that you cannot get sick enough to heal someone else. I get this. But I believe it's something we all have to fight against during a failed relationship.

> Codependency also explains other issues: "Avoiding situations that might cause discomfort or anxiety, much like compulsive gamblers, alcoholics, etc. A set of compulsive behaviors learned by family members in order to adapt in a setting where there is addiction, neglect, physical or emotional abuse, chronic illness or a dysfunction that creates an environment of significant emotional pain and stress. Maladapted: poorly suited to a particular use, purpose, or situation" (Wikipedia).

I'm sure there is way more to it, but the assumed remedy seems to be group counseling, to be with like others, where speaking your mind and standing up for yourself are practiced in a controlled environment, and to learn how to be more assertive and how to value yourself. I can't recall if this was ever offered from my past counselor as I'd never tried it. And I just couldn't seem to appoint blame to my upbringing. I still can't.

Enough of the psychobabble; I'm not a doctor. If you need to know more for the sake of your own health, I recommend you get help from a professional. If you just want more information on it, google it. But don't use the Internet to self-diagnose. You will neurotically find far too many issues relative to your problems.

About 8pm one night, I received a call from Kacey. She was in town, and she wanted to see Thomas. Attempting to avoid this, I told her that he'd be sleeping before nine, so it was not a good time. At about 8:30 p.m., she showed up anyway. In the doorway, I told her that she hadn't done anything according to our custody agreement. I told her that Thomas was already sleeping. She said she just wanted to come in and see him sleeping. She was persistent, and I didn't see any harm in it, so I let her in.

Thomas was sleeping soundly in his crib. I stood next to Kacey for a few minutes. She was smiling, staring down at him. "Don't wake him up," I whispered as I left the room. After about a half hour, I opened the door to my son's room and found Kacey sleeping on the floor next to the crib. I put a blanket on her and closed the door. She looked as though she hadn't slept in a while. Being still highly suspicious of her actions, I decided I had to sleep in front of the door right outside Thomas's room. It was the only way I would get any sleep that night.

I grabbed my sleeping bag and bed down in front of the door.

In the morning, all was well, so I went about my daily routine. Allowing Kacey to sleep in, I stepped over her and proceeded to give Thomas his breakfast and take him to day care for the day. He wouldn't even know she was there.

I went to work. Not expecting her to still be there when I came home for lunch, at noon I found Kacey still sleeping in the same somewhat-awkward position. It had now been about fifteen hours she had been sleeping. Feeling somewhat startled by her stillness, I tried to wake her. She remained in a very deep sleep, where I could move her whole body and she wouldn't even flinch. Finally, after shaking her and raising my voice, she came to.

"What?" she spoke.

"Jesus! Are you okay? You've haven't even moved since nine last night! You're freakin' me out! I was ready to call 911!"

Acting like I just disturbed her nap, she groggily replied, "What time *is* it?"

"Uh, daytime? I assume you haven't slept in a while."

She would gather her purse and jacket and rush out the door. If she was currently in a state of depression, I wouldn't recognize it. In the past, I failed to recognize any of her abnormal behavior. Before life gave me a wake-up call, it would seem I was so selfish that I only had time for those who made me laugh. It wouldn't matter if I did recognize this as depression. She'd made it perfectly clear to me that she was no longer taking my advice.

In a time before caller ID, I began to receive many hung-up calls at any given time of the day. My suspicions would range from

Kacey, Amanda, or possibly one of Kacey's old friends. It wasn't so bad I had to change my number. I just figured it would end soon.

In May, Kacey called late one night. "John?" she asked.

"Yea?" I replied.

After a brief silence, I realized who it was. "Are you okay?" I asked.

"I don't know. I don't know what the hell is going on." Her voice was whispered like she was an abductee. She sounded fragile and secretive, unlike our prior conversations.

"What do you mean? Where are you?" I asked.

Unsure of herself, she replied, "I'm at a pay phone. At some grocery store. I'm with some people. I don't really know what I'm doing here."

"You need to get somewhere where they can help you. You know that, right?" I replied.

"Why? What's the point?" she asked.

"The point is, you haven't seen your son in months. You need help."

"I gotta go. Sorry." She hung up.

> You need to go there without guessing the future.
> You need to go there without guessing.
> You need to go there without.
> You need to go there.
> You need to go.
> You need to.
> You need…
> You.

I told Kacey several months ago, as if it was the only card I held, that if she checked herself in somewhere, I would bring Thomas to see her the day the doctors released her. I would repeatedly remind her of this. Through reading these books on bipolar disorders, or manic depression, these writers, mostly doctors, had me convinced that through the magic of medication, their patients were miraculously changed for the better within months. I'm not saying they can't be, but they shouldn't make you believe that helping them is easy. It's just like one of my favorite old psychology jokes: "How many shrinks does it take to change a lightbulb? Just one, but that lightbulb has to *want* to change."

Through a phone conversation with Kacey's mother, as if there was something she could do, I would reveal this prior phone conversation to her. She told me she hadn't heard much from Kacey but seemed well-informed. She sympathized with me and said she would try and talk with Kacey when possible. Even though we discussed her daughter, she had become someone I confided in on occasion. She offered a few books on the subject so I knew she was well aware of manic depression. She was also wise enough to know that you can't help someone until they want help. I began to notice that I only made her sad when we talked and I shouldn't be revealing anything that would lead her to choose sides. I would lose. I didn't even know what I was trying to win, but I was walking a very fine line by sharing this with her family, like speaking freely to the cops, knowing what you say can and will be held against you. We would be at odds off and on in the future, but Kacey's mother is truly a remarkable person.

I would eventually be informed by the police that the guilty party who stole the prior tenant's identity was not Kacey. It was Amanda and her friend. I was told they were caught on camera returning items to an electronics store for cash. Simply by obtaining his mail and a credit card offer, they were able to acquire a credit card in his name.

I was shocked. Amanda had been my friend and confidant through all the chaos with Kacey. She had been there to take care of Thomas's physical and emotional needs while I was unavailable. I was again baffled by the actions of someone I trusted. I would inform Amanda of my awareness of this news over the phone. She would attempt apologies, but I would refuse to see her or discuss any more of this with her. Later, I would also apologize to Kacey for my accusations. While in the same breath, I would remind her that she did ruin my credit with the other cards.

I could envision what a normal life would be. I would try to pretend to have one, hoping it would actually happen.

At my apartment, Laura, the newly acquired babysitter I met through Amanda, had become a consistent guest. Unlike everyone else in my life, she didn't seem to have any issues; she was too young. She was a senior in high school, eighteen years old. She brought me books from her school library on mental illnesses and information on how to write my own book. She was extremely underpaid as I was about a dollar an hour above qualifying for welfare. Her father was great with kids and had a farm place just outside of town with sheep and ATVs and room to run around. Thomas would often spend time there. I was back playing league basketball and working hard again. My life was becoming somewhat normal. I was truly practicing the adage "Fake it till you make it."

Summer of '95

These were taken from actual journal entries (AJE) from 1995.

I received a phone call from Kacey late at night. (Depression must have finally arrived.) She was crying and apologizing and assuring me that she was going to get better. I told her to just check herself in somewhere. (AJE, June 3, 1995)

Got the call that I always thought I would but it still surprised me. She said we were good together and that if I could see her now, I'd know she was different. I told her she has to keep getting help to see Thomas and she agreed. She said she misses me and Thomas and says she needs a couple months to get it together. She asked to see him after her appointment. I didn't really comment and we said good-bye. She acts like nothing's happened. Who does she think she is? (AJE, June 12, 1995)

From all sides...
(Couldn't locate actual journal entry)

Around June 20th, I received a phone call informing me that Rob was brutally murdered. (Rob, our friend from Kale's and my favorite bar). I was told that Rob's brother, who was known to be in and out of mental hospitals much of his life, was suspected. I attended the funeral but Kale couldn't make the trip.

Several days later, I would find an article in our local paper about manic depression. Amanda's mother had done an interview. Amanda was in jail. It was sometime near the end of June, I received this letter from Amanda:

John,

How are you and Thomas doing? I bet he is getting really big! My mom said that you called her a couple weeks ago—after you read that article in the paper. Pretty nifty huh? Well, now my deep dark secret is out, but I'm kind of relieved. That may sound kind of dumb. Since I have been in here, I have had a lot of time to think. I am twenty-four years old and finally figured out what I don't want. Now all I have to do is figure out what I do want.

A lot of things have changed since I have last talked to you. I guess you could say this is the best thing that happened to me. This has really given me a big dose of reality. For the first time in my life, my eyes have really opened to how bad things have gotten. I can tell you what it was like, and I can tell you what it's like now, but I'm still not sure what happened. Everything just seems like a big blur.

I am truly sorry for anything I have done to hurt you. I really do miss your friendship and hope that someday we can be friends again. You really have a positive influence on me and that is the kind of friends I need now. You may or may not be happy to know that I have cut all ties off with "Bill" and that was very hard for me. You know how I felt about him, but I know that I can't keep on the way we were. I have started to take care of myself. It feels good and I don't want to stop. I have a real long way to go and a lot of things to prove to people that I care about and regain their trust again, but I am going to do it.

I would like to hear from you. I will be here until 8/25, if you want to write. If you don't, I understand! I am truly sorry for any pain I have caused you.

Amanda.

Amanda had since been sentenced to two months in jail for fraud and two years of probation with random testing for medication, Depakote. I would eventually speak to her on the phone, mostly about manic depression. She associated it to the feeling of being high on cocaine—very ambitious and energetic but completely lost. She said her memory was very much affected, and once she even purchased a washer-dryer combination, and when they showed up to install it, she had no memory of the purchase. She admitted that when in this state of mind, no one could bring her back to reality. If they tried, she would run. If cocaine is comparable, I can truly relate. There is nothing that can be offered to meet the equivalent of the experience of euphoria. But just like me, the depression that follows is unbearable.

I wouldn't let Amanda back into my and Thomas's life. I told her that I had to get away from the chaos of the recent past. I thanked her for coming clean with me and wished her luck. I didn't know exactly why I was so upset with Amanda. She didn't steal from me. Apparently, I was just sick of being taken advantage of and lied to, tired of playing the fool. Yeah, I looked out for myself sometimes, if I was not blinded by love.

My estranged relationship with Kacey would continue as usual. She would eventually get counseling and see Thomas on occasion later in the year. I'm not going to speculate any more than I have about her illness as it was quickly becoming none of my business, and perhaps it never was.

CHAPTER 15

Kale

Beware the man who walks alone; for he
hides his hate. His pain is unknown.
He's quick to lash out and strike against
those who laugh in their defense.
It's not your fault that he retains his
hatred and guilt that forever remains.
But it's for your own good that I do warn.
It's revenge he seeks for just being born.
So walk away oh curious one, and
be glad your life is left undone.
Keep your thoughts to your-
self, your opinions unknown.
And beware the man who walks alone.

It was around the Fourth of July 1995. I met up with Kale to go fishing. He informed me of how he was fired from work for punching
his boss. He said, "I grenaded his nose!" I asked for the details, but
at first he was somewhat reluctant. He didn't seem to be too proud
of this.

Eventually, I got him to talk. "What, did you knock him out?"
I asked.

"No. The tough son of a bitch fought back! We were wrestling
when the other guys pulled us apart!"

"Did he have it comin'?"

"I don't know. I think so. No one else seemed to mind," he replied.

He would give more details later on.

This same week, we were away from others and free to speak openly. Thomas was sleeping in the car seat in the back of my Blazer. Kale and I were en route to another lake for fishing as the first one was inactive. (Sometimes we actually tried to catch fish.) It was a rare calm sunshiny day. He asked me if I wanted to hear something crazy. Of course, it's what I do.

Completely sober, he didn't have to tell me to 'be here now'.

In a very casual tone, Kale began, "What if I told ya that a couple guys I met in Cali tried to kill me? Twice!"

"What?"

"Yeah, poison me. I finished my lunch and one of 'em points at my dishes 'n says to the other, 'You believe he ate all that? And nothin's happening?'"

I interrupted, "Ah, sounds to me like they were just fuckin' with ya."

"Possible. But not the second time... The second time I woke up with the same guy holdin' a gun to my face. I got up, and I heard the click of the gun, but it didn't fire. I know he pulled the trigger!"

"You didn't commence to kickin' his ass?" I replied.

"No. Musta been in shock. I just got the hell outta there! I even heard him explainin' it later to his friend when he asked him why he didn't get rid of me. He told him, 'I tried! Fuckin' gun misfired. Didn't go off!'"

I replied, "Who the hell are these guys, and why would they want to kill you?"

He continued, "These guys work for some drug dealer. I know they got ties to the mafia. You can't repeat this shit, you know!"

"I know."

"They think I know shit that I didn't really know until this happened. They think I know about their boss's son killing someone. They're trying to get rid of me in case I go to the cops."

"Well, did you know about the boss's kid?"

"No. But I put it all together. I know now."

"Why don't you go to the cops?" I asked.

"I don't trust 'em. That's prolly the quickest way to gettin' killed."

"What the hell are you supposed to do now?" I asked.

"I don't know. I get the feeling that their boss told 'em to leave me alone. That I'm not gonna narc on anyone. Maybe he thinks I'm good luck for him because I dodged death twice."

"So you just gonna wait and see what happens?"

"Yeah. I'm gonna keep my mouth shut. I'm only tellin' you 'cause I trust ya. I'm thinkin' I'm gonna get a payoff for this."

Kale had often told me creative stories that exploited my naivety. He'd draw out a story as far as possible until I'd say, "All right, fuck you!" Then he'd bust out in laughter. I was gullible, but I could usually spot his fabrications before they went too far. This time, I was confused.

After I attempted to absorb this story, I checked to see his poker face. I sensed nothing, but I threw out the bullshit flag anyway. "So how long you gonna drag this story out?"

"Why? What do you think about it?"

"It sounds to me like you got this out of a book or a movie."

Staring out the window, lowering his voice, he proclaimed, "Not this time, Johnny."

My senses became instantly enhanced. Even now I can remember this exact location, the sound of the tires rolling over the gravel, the warm breeze blowing through my window, and the way Kale told such a serious, effective story in such a nonchalant manner. My memory is impacted so dramatically at this moment because part of me knew this to be the beginning of the end of what innocence we had left. I didn't know enough about anything to make a judgment. I'd heard many similar stories, but something was different about this one. And my logical and intelligent best friend was beginning to behave like a stranger. I didn't know why he would want me to believe this if it wasn't true.

The rest of the day continued as normal. At times, I would make a few inquiries about his story, but he'd brush me off or tell me that it was complicated and then change the subject, and that I already knew more that I should. I would bring Thomas to my parents and meet up with Kale later that night.

I wouldn't inquire about his prior story until we were parting ways later that night. He told me to forget about it. That I was right—he made it up. He got it all out of a book. But before he left, he asked, "What would you say if it was true?"

So as not to look like a played fool, I replied, "Well, I'd tell you that you're either losin' your mind or you're in a shitload of trouble."

Within the next week, Kale and I would have another 'be here now' moment. He proceeded to tell me that the story he had given me before was not taken from a book. He said that it really happened and was still happening. He gave me more of the details. He would describe everything, from their leather jackets to what type of gun they had tried to use. Likely thinking of my safety, he would leave out any clues as to whom they were or where they were from, saying that they were just a couple of drinking buddies (biker dudes) he'd gotten high with a few times. He said they were now getting along. They would tell him that they could get him anything he wanted.

I had no reason not to believe him. Out of all the stories he'd shared with me about his life on the road, I never questioned the validity. He was not one to intentionally attempt to impress others, specifically me. If he was telling me a story while a witness was in the room, the witness would always collaborate. And often they would add more ridiculous details that Kale forgot. I normally found these stories hilarious. This time, I was worried. We made light of every situation in our lives thus far. There was absolutely no humor in this one.

I would like to believe I had asked all the proper questions. Kale continued to think that he should just keep quiet and he would get paid off someday. I asked how he knew about getting paid off. "Who was telling you about the money and what to do next? How are you communicating with these people?"

> "The truth is stranger than fiction. Fiction is obligated to stick to possibilities, truth isn't."
> (Scott Fitzgerald).

Kale then asked me if I thought it was possible to implant a radio receiver in someone's head and be able to speak to that person form far away. (Instantly, my heart sunk. I had just finished reading about manic depression and schizophrenia. The one sure thing I remembered was that hearing voices and having delusions is the basic definition of schizophrenia. Not yet willing to pin that label on Kale, I kept listening, hoping there was some other explanation. We continued our conversation.)

I said I had never heard of implanting receivers or chips in someone apart from science fiction movies and books. He tried to convince me by pointing out the technology we now had and what had likely been done by our government without our knowledge. I said that it might be possible but kept asking him why he was adamant about knowing. He told me that he thought someone may have implanted one in the back of his head because he was hearing live voices and didn't have any other explanation for it. I instantly tried to debunk this idea. I told him that even if they could, why they would do that to him? What would make him so special that they would go through so much trouble just for him? He couldn't say for sure but said it was the way they could keep tabs on every move he made. He went on to say that he punched his boss because of these voices.

He said he was up in a lift with a tool partner when he felt sick and asked to be brought down to the ground. His work partner obliged. Kale proceeded to walk right over to the boss and give him a heavy right hand. He went on to tell me that the voices didn't actually tell him to assault his boss; they just told him that he was in on the deal. Kale stated, "So I guess punchin' him was *my* decision."

Instead of blatantly telling him he was crazy, because I was not qualified to make that judgment, I told him I didn't really believe him about these voices and asked him if he had been doing any heavy drugs. He told me what I believed at the time to be true: that he hadn't been trippin' on acid or doing anything other than smoking weed and drinking since last winter. Kale, in his own investigation, also felt that maybe someone had hypnotized him while he was drunk or high and put these ideas in his head.

Somewhat afraid to know more, I wouldn't continue my inquiry of his drug use. I didn't know enough about drug use and its connection to mental illnesses to comment any further. I told myself to just listen.

I did tell him that I read about this in some of the books I was reading while trying to understand manic depression. I told him that I felt this was a mental illness called paranoid schizophrenia. He said he'd heard about that before but believed this was way too real to be his imagination.

The next few times I saw Kale, he continued to act very paranoid and constantly talked about death and paybacks. At one point, he told me that his sister, his mother, and the people that he used to work with were all in on this. He said most couldn't remember because they had been hypnotized or given a certain pill that could make them forget. He talked about how the voices were always testing people. He said they would put the people in the front of a room and interrogate them until they confessed to everything.

He began to openly share these twisted thoughts with his family. At one point, he told his sister that when he was at the bank, he asked the voices if they could show him a mental picture of the clerk naked. He said that when he closed his eyes, they showed him. He said the power these people had was phenomenal. He sometimes laughed about what they would tell him.

There were times when he would also disregard the severity of this situation. We would be fishing, and he would seem as normal as could be, then without any warning to his thoughts, he would tell me that it probably wasn't safe for Thomas to stand next to him in case someone was across the lake with a sniper rifle. They might miss him and hit Thomas. I would respond by telling him to keep his morbid thoughts to himself as I secretly began to question the safety of my own son. I didn't fear Kale, but just the thought of such an act repulsed me, and I still didn't know how much was true and what was imaginary. Kale would at times, apologize and shake his head in disgust of his own words. And in his anger over his current state of mind, he mentioned that if these people didn't pay him off at the end, he was going to seek revenge for the hell they were putting him through.

I began to insist that he get help. From what I knew about schizophrenia, which wasn't much at the time, the only relief was medication.

Our time together soon became taxing as he continued to express his negative thoughts—about how wrong people were about their lives and how some of our longtime friends were not whom they appeared to be. Although he expressed great insight, I would have to stand up for our friends, and we would inadvertently spend much of this time arguing. The fun we used to have had quickly turned into heated discussions about philosophy, life, and death. I told him, "You're scaring your family, scaring me." Kale recognized this, and at the end of one of our evenings, standing outside with his hands on the open window of my car door, he submissively leaned down and said, "You believe me. Don't ya, Johnny?"

"I believe that you believe it," I answered.

"Good enough," he replied.

It had been less than two weeks since he brought this to my attention. On the thirteenth of July, Kale's sister Tanya, Tanya's daughter, Joan, and Thomas and I all went fishing together. It started off as normal as usual. Then I noticed Kale not fishing, not even attempting to. He wrapped himself up in a sleeping bag, covering his entire body. It was about eighty degrees outside. A few hours in, when he was up and about, he began making strange offensive and morbid comments about death and betrayal. The kids were close enough to hear him, so I motioned for Tanya to take them for a walk. Feeling confident with Joan in agreement, I began to confront Kale about his behavior. There would be no more dancing around this subject. I told him that we were all sick of hearing this shit. Laying it all on the line, I told him that his whole story is bullshit. That no one was trying to kill him, that there was no money, and that his family and I have had it with this crazy talk. I went on to say I was going to call the cops to come and pick him up and take him to a mental hospital if he continued to talk like this. He slowly moved in to look me in the eyes. With the look he only used to give his enemies, he stated, "Try it!"

Joan moved in between us and thankfully defused the situation. I had found his breaking point. I was glad his family backed me up, but being the way Kale was, I was no way going to push him any further. At the end of the day, I shook his hand, and in my most sincere tone, I told him that if things were to really get out of hand, that he should come find me. We'd go together. I had mentioned many times that we needed to see a professional. It was the only way I knew how to stop the voices.

I returned home. I called Dr. Benet (Kacey and Amanda's former doctor). I informed him about Kale. He told me that it sounded exactly like schizophrenia and that I should bring him immediately. I told the doctor that he likely couldn't afford to see him at his hospital, but I would try to get him to go somewhere. He told me that he would likely need inpatient treatment, but I shouldn't hesitate to take him somewhere—not tomorrow, but now. I understood the weight of the issue but was hesitant because you just don't tell Kale what to do. I thanked him for the advice and said I'd try my best.

Two nights later, Kale called me from a nearby motel, "Hey man! You told me to call you if things got worse! Well..., it's not good!"

"Why? What's up?" I ask. "What's happening?"

"I don't want to talk about it on the phone," he answers. "Can you come here?"

"Why? What the hell is going on? Where are you?"

"I'm at that sixth street motel, room 12... They're starting to come through the TV now! What the hell am I gonna do?"

"Hold on!" I respond. "I'll be there in a few minutes."

I arrive at his room and knock on the door. He cautiously peaks through the curtains, opens the door, steps out to take a suspicious look around, and then motions for me to come in. Contrary to his usual cocky display of self-confidence, he looks exhausted and uneasy. He sits down on the end of the bed. Staring at the TV, he takes a gulp of his beer. Calmly, I ask what the problem is. He hesitates. With the hand that's gripping the beer, he points at the TV and through a casual, yet affirming voice he declares, "The things I used to hear in my head are now coming through the TV and through the radio in my car."

Aware of his recent condition, I point at his beer and say, "Do you think you should be drinkin?"

"Ah", he shrugs, "seems to keep 'em quiet."

As I pause in search of a proper response, we are both reminded of our familiarity during this brief, uncomfortable silence. Recognizing my hesitation and before I could speak, he looks up to say, "Look, man. This is not my imagination! Either these people are really fuckin with me now or I am completely losing my mind. I think it's time we go find out if I'm really fuckin crazy!" He makes eye contact once again and with that unyielding stare I've known most of my life, he asks, "You up for it?"

I almost knew this time was coming. I gave him hope that there was something that could be done, and now here we were. I told Kale that we needed to go to the hospital tonight. He insisted we would go in the morning, telling me he'd pay for me to miss work and for gas. I told him to promise me we'd leave in the morning, and he agreed. I decided to accept a beer and sit down to listen to some more details.

He went on to say that the voices were now constant and becoming stronger. They also told him he should listen to me. He was told that there was an old guy, a friend from Kale's past, who was experiencing everything that he was; every time he drank, the old man got drunk. Every time he smoked weed, the old man got high. He chuckled and said the old man was having a blast but couldn't take the wear and tear on his body anymore, so he had to stop.

I asked what happened to the voices when he drank. He said that whenever he got drunk, the voices would get hard to understand. He felt that by getting them drunk, he wouldn't have to listen to them.

"When did they get stronger?" I asked.

"The last few days." He went on, "I asked 'em if this was God. They laughed at me!"

I took the next day off. I called my boss in the morning. Whether it was due to my depression or my son with the flu, I'd almost always had an excuse for missing work and was sick of myself for calling in yet again, so this time I decided to tell the truth. "I have to take my friend to the hospital. He's hearing voices." There would be no need for further explanation. That morning, Kale and I headed for the hospital. We picked up a twelve-pack for the road.

Kale had always been the first to say "Bullshit" when someone told an unbelievable story. I'd been listening to his advice my entire life. I didn't know of anyone who shared his ability to simplify a problem and to be as rational in defining it. I'd always thought of him as extremely advanced in determining what should be thought about and what should go left unanswered. Now here I was trying to convince him of trusting me and my advice. And if I'd ever had any question about the legitimacy of a mental illness, it was suddenly and boldly staring me in the face.

On the way there, I shouldn't have, but I asked a lot of questions. Kale seemed to be in a fairly good mood. I was somewhat hoping that after his trip to the hospital, he might forget some of what was currently happening. Part of me thought if he talked about this enough, maybe he'd recognize it as separate from who he was. If he could see himself from the outside, maybe he'd be more apt to comply with the doctor.

At first, Kale didn't seem to mind my questions. When he again mentioned being paid off for keeping their secrets, I asked how much. "Well, they offered me a million. But I told them that the Bible says we are punished seven times over for our sins, so I asked for seven million."

"Where do they get this money?"

"Well, apparently, gettin' rid of that guy made 'em some serious money. So it sounds like they're gonna give it to me. They also said they'd taken some out as hush money for other people involved." He went on, "They gave me a set of numbers that I have to remember for when it's all over. I think it's for a lock box."

"They can tell you this shit at any time? Are they saying anything right now?" I asked.

Before he could answer, I leaned in to put my ear to his. "What the fuck you doin?" he asked, pushing me away.

"Well, if there's some kind of receiver in your head, maybe I can hear it too?" I was not trying to be a wiseass. I didn't think before I did it. I did this as a reaction. Maybe part of me wanted to show him that his theory wasn't possible. Before he could comment on my actions, I asked, "What the hell do you think they want? Why would they fuck with you all day?"

"They're just constantly testing me. They always want me to prove whatever I'm thinking." He paused. "Ya know, just shut up for a while. You know too much already. You realize they once told me that you were in on this."

"What?" I replied. "How the hell is that possible?"

"They told me you knew something but held out on me for my own good. They said you were lookin' out for me. I told them that we've been friends a long time."

After I let that sink in, I cautiously asked, "What else have they said about me?"

Laughing, he said, "Well, they once thought you were gay."

"What?"

Laughing harder, he said, "Yeah, it's true."

"Whatever."

"Ha-ha ... Well, they wondered why you hang out with me all the time. I told 'em that you are a little different, but you just have trouble with women."

"Yeah, true," I replied. After a long pause, I could still hear him snickering.

Defensively, I declared, "Well, I'm glad you cleared that up with them. I wouldn't want some millionaire drug lord from California thinkin' I was gay!"

The laughter stopped. With his finger in my face and tension on his, he angrily asked me, "Hey! You think I'm makin' this shit up?"

"No, I don't. But I don't know how the hell you find it funny."

"Yeah, yeah. Just shut the fuck up for a while."

We continued with our beers.

After several miles, staring out the window, Kale asked, "What makes you so sure they can take the voices away?"

"I'm not sure. But from everything I've read, it's the only option."

"Well, I hope so." Making his hand into the shape of a gun, he pointed it under his chin as he continued, "Cause if they don't, it's gonna be this for me!"

Pushing his hand away, I replied, "Knock it off! They're gonna help you. You gotta see that." I tried to lighten the mood. "You care if I write a book about this?"

"Go ahead. If I end up killin' these fuckers and gettin' their money, you can call it *Reverse*. No, wait. Call it *Revenge* and spell it backward. That'd be a cool cover."

"Well, I'm gonna write somethin'. This is crazy shit!" I replied.

A few miles before town, we were approaching a cop. He had someone pulled over. Kale said, "Part of me wants you to just stop and tell this cop everything I know."

"Not now," I replied. "We're drinkin'!"

We arrived in town. Kale wanted to hit a bar before we'd go in because he figured they were going to keep him for a while once he was inside. We did a couple shots, had a couple more beers, and kept our conversation light, with me doing most of the talking as I was feeling fairly drunk. I was expecting to be laughing hard at something soon, just like we'd always done. But sadly, since the voices arrived, this was now a rare occurrence. Not really knowing how our former outbursts of laughter began, we now had no means to retrieve it.

By the time we arrived at this state-funded hospital, I was feeling it. I worried that they might call the cops when they would see us walk in. I mentioned this to Kale. He said, "These guys are above cops. They're not gonna bust ya. You're takin your friend to the nuthouse!"

We walked in. Kale walked away to talk with a receptionist and a doctor for just a few minutes while I found some water to drink. He returned and sat down. As we waited, typical of a mental hospital, they hauled someone in wearing a strait jacket, kicking and screaming. With a raised eyebrow, Kale and I shared a concerned look.

Eventually, a doctor came outside where Kale and I were having a cigarette. He asked a little about what was happening. He asked Kale if it was okay to continue to ask him a series of questions while in my presence. Kale confirmed. He asked him if he could name the last five presidents. Searching for the answer in my mind, I quickly realized that I couldn't answer. Kale correctly answered rather easily. He then asked him what day it was and where he was. He again answered correctly. He then asked him to repeat the same five words in the order that the doctor would say them. The words have nothing in common—for example, *train, cereal, sky, notebook,* and *dollar.* Kale could only repeat a few. He asked him a couple of small multiplication problems. Kale answered with ease. Then he asked how many nickels were in two dollars. After several seconds, Kale couldn't answer. He shook his head in his own disgust. After the doctor left, Kale and I discussed the questions.

Laughing, I said, "Damn, I'm glad he didn't ask me anything! I'd be right in here with ya!"

Knowing me well, Kale responded, "Well, I bet it wouldn't hurt ya!"

The doctor then came back and asked Kale to accompany them to another room while gesturing for me to sit in the waiting area. Before long, I was out. Kale's doctor woke me up about an hour later, saying, "How are you doing by the way?"

Coming to, I told him, "It's been a wild ride, Doc!"

As he poured me some coffee, he informed me that Kale was going to stay and asked me to sign to be his emergency contact. Kale and I shook hands as he gave me a sincere "Thank you." He told me he'd call me in a week.

Kale would later call me to tell me he received an MRI scan. They didn't find any physical damage. I was hoping they would. I wanted Kale to have a tangible reason for this chaos—something he could understand and tolerate.

CHAPTER 16

Fallen Angel

The following weekend, Kale called and wanted to be picked up. I was fairly surprised but told him I would. Tanya would come with me. It was a Saturday. We arrived at the gate where Kale was standing with his duffel bag, looking like a true transient. His face was emotionless. He didn't respond to us when we greeted him. He threw his bag in the back and got in. Upon pulling away, when I looked in the backseat, he had the look of Jack Nicholson from *One Flew Over the Cuckoo's Nest*. He was staring straight ahead, attempting to cross his eyes. Tanya and I exchanged a questionable look. Finally, he couldn't contain himself and let out a belly laugh, making me jump as he slapped the back of my seat. "Ha-ha! What's the matter with you guys?"

Relieved, I replied, "Jesus, man. You gotta fuck with us even now?"

"Aw, c'mon. Can't I have a little fun with ya?" he replied.

We pulled away. A few blocks down the road, Tanya asked him what his doctors said. "What's the issue?"

He responded in a serious tone, "Well, ya know when you're watching football on TV, and all the players get in their little circle, you know, their huddle?" We nodded in agreement. Pointing to himself, he said, "Well, I think they're talkin' about *me*!"

We all laughed out loud, though we didn't settle for his answer. He would eventually give us as much information as he wanted to without ever saying the word *schizophrenia*. He went on to say that they gave him some legal drugs and he was supposed to return in a week. This answer would suffice.

Against our recently found better judgment, we would stop at a bar on the way home. Tanya had made arrangements to meet a couple of friends of hers whom she hadn't seen in some time on our way back. When I told Kale this, he argued with me. He wanted to go straight home. I told him to just be a passenger for once, that I was tired of him always calling the shots, that we wouldn't take that long, and that he should just sit back and ride along. We argued for a minute, up to the point where he threatened to kick my ass. I gave him the usual, "Oh yeah, use violence to get your way again!" He decided to fight with harsh words, the way I did, and told me that he was sick of my fakey personality. That I was just as fucked up in the head as he was. I told him, "I'm going to a counselor, just like you are, so yeah, I guess we're both fucked up."

"Well...good!" he replied. With both of us now quietly laughing over our exchange, we exited my Blazer. We settled on that to be the end of our discussion.

While sitting at the bar, Kale drinking a Coke, he placed his cigarettes on the bar. A stranger sitting next to him asked, "Why do your cigarettes have your name taped on them?"

Eyeing up the stranger, Kale answered, "Well, they do that for you when you've either been in the hospital or in jail."

I intervened, "Yeah, you got any more dumb questions?"

The stranger walked away. We would arrive home in a couple of hours.

> Kacey's (new) psychiatrist, Dr. "Houseman" called and asked if he could schedule an appt. with me to discuss Kacey. It was done. (AJE, August 3, 1995)

Why not? Free counseling. I was engrossed in the world of psychiatry: Kale, Kacey, Amanda, and the circumstances surrounding the death of the bartender, Rob. I would love to be able to gain information that would benefit someone.

At this appointment, the doctor explained that he had received a letter from Kacey's mother containing some of Kacey's history. He asked many questions about our time together, and I answered as best I could. I also told him that she was once, rather hastily, diagnosed as bipolar, or manic depressive. I eventually asked why he wanted to see me. He told me that she had missed her last two appointments and was wondering if I could help him get her back in ... Me?

Much of August carried on the same. I went fishing with Kale for a couple of weekends. He was quieter now as I decided not to bring up anything about the recent past. He was taking his medication. He would slowly sip on a beer while fishing. A six-pack seemed to take him all day. He would still make bizarre comments at times and talk about our favorite bartender, Rob, and how he was murdered. It was obvious that this aforementioned tragedy bothered him. Not only because he lost a great friend, but the way in which it happened—to consider what those who are losing touch with reality are sometimes capable of.

Sometime in September, Kale checked himself back in to the hospital on his own for a couple of weeks to adjust his medication and possibly, in his words, to dry out. Joan, Tanya, and I came for a visit. A counselor would take Joan and Tanya aside to talk while Kale began to show me the facilities. He also wanted to show me his room. We asked for permission to enter the dorm room area, and although it was not normal procedure, I was allowed down the hall. Before we arrived at Kale's room, we were approached by a large man dressed in a robe. He aggressively walked up to me and while in my face, he asked, "Are you here to see me? Are you one of them? You know what goes on in here?"

Kale interrupted, "Hey, Jim! Check it out." Holding up a match from a matchbook, he continued, "Look what I got!"

The weary stranger smiled, took the match, proceeded to dig it into his own ear, and silently walked away. Kale turned to me. "Yeah, lotta fuckin' weirdos in here. You can't let your guard down."

I saw many people sitting in silence, staring out the window. I made some stupid derogatory comment. Kale interrupted, "Hey! They're not dumb. They're just thinkin' about somethin' else."

Continuing down the hall, the more alert and respondent patients all waved and said "Hey, Kale!" while he walked by. He peaked in at a couple of rooms to introduce me to his friends while describing their illnesses. As they would turn to look, Kale would say, "This is Mike, he's schizophrenic. There's Doug, he's depressed."

When we entered Kale's room, his roommate was sitting at a desk. As he turned around, Kale addressed him. "Here's Stan, he's just fuckin angry!"

Stan stood up and replied "Fuck you!" as he left the room. It seemed Kale was the hall boss.

Kale then reached up and grabbed a ceramic eagle off the shelf that he had painted in art class. He handed it to me. "Here's for helpin' me with all this crazy shit!"

At a loss for words, "Thanks" was all I could say.

He would walk me back out to the yard where Tanya and Joan were waiting. I would leave the three of them with the doctor to talk.

I could tell that Kale didn't know why he was with such strange people. I didn't know either. There are many who sat in their chairs for hours and just mumbled and moaned. Some struggled to hold their heads up, likely due to heavy medication. Some of them could hardly hold a conversation. I was sure he felt like an outcast, but in typical Kale fashion—if at first you don't feel comfortable in your surroundings, force others to conform to your comfort. He was so good at making himself at home.

> Saw Kale. He still can't understand what is wrong with him. I feel sorry for him. The whole place freaks me out. Why would God let such a thing happen to people? No calls from Kacey. (AJE, September 24, 1995)

Kale would eventually go home to his mother's. We spoke on the phone often, but I was also seeing a counselor and decided that drinking was not helping me with anything. Not knowing how to behave in public without it, I was forced to withdraw to my apartment. I was also low on cash.

I began to show more interest in Thomas's babysitter, Laura. I hardly had enough money to pay her, but she kept showing up even when I didn't need a sitter. I realized she was too young for me and that I was still emotionally unavailable, but Thomas and I truly enjoyed her company. She made me feel normal. She was well aware of all my current situations and was a very good listener. She read my poems and continued to entice me to write a book about these recent issues. She believed in me.

Fall was now upon us, and our weather was beginning to change. Kacey would reappear at her appointments off and on and would have her doctor call me and tell me that he didn't see any reason she couldn't see her son. He recommended supervised visits. I reported to Kacey that she was now welcome anytime, but she wouldn't be able to have him overnight until my lawyer received the necessary paperwork.

Kale and I had been out a couple of times recently, and he seemed to be doing well. We wouldn't discuss much of this recent past. He seemed to be feeling better, and I wasn't going to disturb. It was now pheasant season. Kale called and wanted to go hunting. We did this often. I would turn down the offer. I mentioned how broke I was, that Laura was here with Thomas, and that I shouldn't be out drinking and fucking around—that I'm trying to get my life in order. We talked for a while on the phone as he mentioned that he might go visit his son instead. He'd been seeing Daniel off and on for the past year, but he and Rachel would often end up in arguments. He was drinking often several months ago, so she likely didn't want him around. I don't know if he openly spoke about his illness with her. Before hanging up with him, I asked Kale if the medication he was on had taken the voices away. He said, "Naw, they just shut 'em up for a while."

On Friday, October 27, 1995, I received a phone call from Joan. She asked me if I had seen Kale. I hadn't, but I told her I had spoken to him last weekend on the phone when he had asked me to go hunting with him. Through our further discussion, we agreed that he may be up north visiting Daniel. She told me to call her the next time I'd see him. I told her I would do so. We hung up. Concerned, I called her back a few minutes later and told her to do the same. The next night I left Thomas with my parents and went out, hoping to run into Kale.

I drank alone. I stopped at a couple of secluded bars by the lake where Kale and I had recently been. After several hours, I made my way to a friend's who also lived in that area. She wasn't home that night, but I'd been drinking way too much to continue driving, so I, unintentionally, spent the rest of the night in my car in her driveway. In the morning, the Taylors were on my way to my parents' home, so I stopped in to see if Kale was there or if they had heard from him. Joan was still sleeping, so I sat down to talk with Tanya. She too believed that Kale was visiting his son.

After about a half hour, a policeman knocked on the door. He asked to speak to Kale's mother. Tanya awakened Joan. We all went to the door. Three officers were standing outside. One was wearing a suit.

"Joan?" he asked.

"Yes?" she answered.

"I hate to have to tell you, but Kale was found dead this morning at Lake Alvin from a shotgun wound to the head."

With her hand over her mouth, she uttered, "No!"

He proceeded to give us only a few details about this discovery. He said he was found by a group of hunters and that he would give us more information as the investigation would continue.

They left. Joan and Tanya looked at me. Searching for words, I said, "I fucking knew it! He told me on the way to the hospital. If they didn't take the voices away…"

We walked around in silence. There was absolutely nothing we could do now. I told them I had to go and that I would call them tonight. I continued to my parents' home to pick up my son. When I first saw my son, I immediately thought of how Kale began his conversations with Thomas. Thomas would find Kale sitting on the couch and harmlessly drop a book on his lap while climbing on to sit next to him. Before Kale began to read to him, he would ask Thomas, "Are you my friend?" To which Thomas would distinctly and so innocently reply "Yes."

I would go on tell my parents what had happened. My mother cried. She rarely cries.

> Was at Kale's this morning. Kale was found dead at the lake. From a shotgun wound to the head. His car was stuck. A dead mink was found on the hood. His body was in the water. They haven't found the gun yet. They didn't say if there was a note. I don't know what happened. He talked about life and death sometimes, but not more than anyone else. (Not more than me.) I just think he would have told me. He was my best friend. I was his. He told me everything. On the way to treatment, he told me that if they didn't take the voices away, he would. I don't know if it's because I'm 'ill' and can't express my feelings, or if I'm still in shock. I can't feel anything. (AJE, October 29, 1995, Sunday)

I tried to go to work the following day. I told my foreman about the situation in the morning. By break time, I'd had enough. I couldn't function. I decided to go to Taylors'. While there, the police showed up with the gun. They found it in the water. When they stood outside on the steps holding the gun and giving more details, all I could think of was how perfectly Kale sawed off the gun barrel to make it easier to handle. Kale and I would often compete over who was the better craftsman. I could picture him saying, "Look at that perfect cut!" I would quickly chase those strange thoughts away.

Kale's brother Steve had received the news and had just returned from California. We all went to the morgue together to witness his body. (I assume they wanted us to see proof so we could begin to grieve.) Kale's weight had been fluctuating lately, and he was heavier now than he used to be. He looked softer and less rigid and athletic, like he had deflated and finally relaxed. I saw his old scars on his knuckles from hard labor and his past fights. I saw his tattoo of an eagle on his arm. It wore the name "Fallen Angel". I saw the gunshot wound. We were told that he walked out into the water, neck-deep, I assumed, to be thorough; to make sure there was no way of surviving. Steve would ask if there was water in his lungs. The mortician quietly replied, "Some." At twenty-eight years old, my best friend, Kale, would remain forever young.

To my best friend,

I was given an eagle, from you my best friend, one month before your life came to an end.

At the time I didn't know how much this had meant.

Much like the price you had paid for the time you had spent.

To make sure I could last in this world, alone. It was your duty and you let it be known.

You told me to get help in case you were gone.

Because you knew of my life and you knew it was wrong.

You made sure of my future, that I could forget the past.

And you wouldn't leave until you knew it at last.

That I would be fine as I went on my way, because you knew somehow I'd have to forgive that day.

You'll always be something more than my friend, because our lives were shared to the very end.

So I thank you for this, dear friend of mine. And I hope you know that within my time.

I will change my life and you can be sure, that this world will know you as great as you were.

Good-bye, best friend.

Saw Kale. They found the gun in the water. The barrel was sawed off. I went with Steve to the spot. It's hitting me now. Thomas is with friends-too stressful. My biggest problem is that he didn't tell me. Not exactly. I thought I was a better friend than that. Did he do it because the voices told him to, or did he not hear the voices, faced reality, and was scared for his family and friends? I want to know his final thoughts. Didn't he know how bad this would hurt? Nothing he ever did alive could cause as much pain. (AJE, October 30)

After viewing the sight at the lake, I played out his last hours. It was a very serene and isolated place. It faced west to view the sunset. Out of all the places we'd been, surrounding the lakes nearby, we were never at this one together. At least, I had never known about it. He would get his car stuck on purpose—no turning back. I can't imagine how many times he was here. The front of the car was facing the water. Elvis gospel music was last played in his tape deck. An empty six-pack was behind his seat. I understand the dead mink on the hood to not be some strange message but to make sure his gun was working properly and maybe to remind others of how he loved to hunt and trap. What thoughts were going on in his mind is something I'll never know and likely never want to know as I have never been quite this close to the end.

Tanya would call me later that night and tell me he did leave a note. It was on the seat. The cops kept this for a couple of days for reasons unknown. I think they were letting our grief pace itself.

I read the note. I was relieved. His words were just like he spoke, short but truthful.

Kale apologized and told his family he loved them. He said he was afraid he was going to hurt somebody; that he misses his brother, Daniel. He'd also written, "Song-Daniel" on his note. He did say, "Me and God are okay." He also left a personal side note for his uncle that would be written on his tombstone.

Continued. That note, and that song (Daniel, by Elton John) have put a certain peace in my heart and in my head. Thank God. I thought the worst was yet to come. Steve, Tanya, Kale's mother and I talked for a while before I left. We talked about God and heaven. Kale's mother is amazing. Tanya is feeling better. Steve is still mad but getting better. Kale is at peace, and so am I. (AJE, October 31)

AJE 11/1 Wed. Went to Taylors' home. Went shopping with Steve and Tanya. I've decided not to say anything at the funeral. (Had contemplated saying a few words at the funeral, but I thought about what Kale would say and I realized I don't have to prove my friendship to anyone). I got to tell Steve a little about schizophrenia and Kale. He didn't say much but agreed about people messing with him also. God I hope I'm wrong about Steve. After reading Kale's note, I told the family about Kale's final thoughts. (In my opinion, anyway). I think we're going to play 'Daniel' at the funeral. They approved. That song is short, but opposite in meaning. It makes me cry and it also makes me smile. I am nervous about tomorrow. What words can come to me now? Tomorrow, I bury my best friend.

I would inform Kacey of Kale's death. Not to provoke sympathy but to hopefully get her to believe in the frailty of sanity. That sometimes you have to admit you are not in control and you need help. Again, she didn't really want to discuss this. She blamed Kale's mindset on a bad childhood and drug use. Of course, she didn't know him near as well as I did, yet I couldn't tell her she's wrong. She was far too intelligent to walk around uninformed, and she'd been to a counselor occasionally. Her opinions still mattered to me.

I didn't notice the normal signs. Maybe I was too close to notice. Kale must have made this decision long ago. We went out together a couple of times recently, and he wouldn't bring up the voices or complain of any trouble. It is how many people who have accepted their fate tend to act when they've made up their mind about suicide. They seem to be at peace with this secretive decision as it also must distract those close to them just enough to believe they are feeling okay. I would learn that he even visited a few old friends and returned a few items he had borrowed, tying up loose ends. Kale and I did share a couple of moments that reminded me of our youth during his last weeks. Just a day of doing what we always did—fishing, reminiscing, and sharing philosophy.

At the funeral, I was not a pallbearer. I sat with the family. I tried to answer many questions this day. I only revealed my opinions to those who knew Kale well; others were likely afraid to ask. Kale did confide in a few close friends and relatives as they had heard other versions of Kale's last few months. His stories were not all the same. (I wrote what I could perceive of his explanation to hearing voices. Kale's applied reasoning did vary, and I was well aware of this. No one searched harder to find the truth behind his illness than he did. What's written is the version I understood.)

I would pin a tiny angel on the shirt of Daniel, Kale's son—the angel on your shoulder. He was just a boy. I didn't have the words then, and I don't have them now. There aren't any.

> Nothing gold can stay.
> Nature's first green is gold, her hardest hue to
>   hold.
> Her early leaf's a flower; but only so an hour.
> The leaf subsides to leaf. So Eden sank to grief.
> So dawn goes down to day. Nothing gold can
>   stay.
>
> (Robert Frost)

This should be the end. I should be done. I will use mostly journal entries to finish as I struggle for the words.

Schizophrenia: a mental disorder often characterized by abnormal social behavior and failure to recognize what is real. Common symptoms include false beliefs, unclear or confused thinking, auditory hallucinations, reduced social engagement and emotional expression, and inactivity. Diagnosis is based on observed behavior and the person's reported experiences. (Wikipedia)

CHAPTER 17

War

> The key to immortality is first liv-
> ing a life worth remembering.
>
> —Bruce Lee

I miss him.
Forever is lost in yesterday's pain
As I desperately hold on to the
knowledge I've gained.
Undecided are my dreams,
unchosen are my words
And the image enlarges of a sight, absurd.
Engulfed in my imagination, be
it worse than the truth
As I long for the ignorance I
enjoyed with youth.
Death has a name, given to some.
Aloud in your ears, until it grows numb.
I miss him.

A friend of Kale's and mine would call me at my apartment. She too had recently suffered a great loss. Whatever her words were, I finally sat down on my kitchen floor while on the phone and began to cry—to cry real tears. An hour later, I felt better. So this is what it's like to feel normal, to grieve, to feel sadness for a legitimate reason.

Steve was now home from California. He was debating on returning to work or staying home for the winter. I was still spending much of my time with the Taylors.

> "Dan" called. (Dan, our mutual childhood friend; Kale's former and Steve's current boss.) He told me about how suspicious Steve was of everyone and how he has withdrawn from everyone; the first signs of paranoid schizophrenia. We talked for a couple hours. Dan is worried. (AJE November 3, 1995, Friday, one day after Kale's funeral)
>
> [I] Rode snowmobile with my brother. Felt pretty good. Haven't heard from Kacey since last Tuesday when I told her about Kale. (When) She said she was real sorry. A minute later, she said she'd see me on Thursday (funeral). I told her not to come and to just stay away for a couple weeks. She wanted to go to the funeral with me and everything. I told her that Kale shot himself because he couldn't stop the mental illness. She said that Kale had a very bad childhood and that was why. She was trying to keep off mental illnesses. (AJE, November 4, 1995, Saturday)

I continued to see a counselor on occasion, when affordable, and was beginning to deal with Kale's death. Looking at my journal, I can tell that I was still overly concerned with Kacey, whether it was lingering love or fear. Although actual depression had yet to be introduced to me, I was learning more about codependency and that I was feeding my old habits by interfering in her life. I began to change a few things about myself and tried to start minding my own business. In doing so, the anxiety that I felt about Thomas's future with his mother had begun to lessen. I was still struggling with work. I also spent much of my time learning more about schizophrenia and trying to explain it to Kale's friends and relatives, many of whom would rather believe in some conspiracy. I wanted to offer them some peace of mind.

Kacey would see a counselor, tell me about it, and then she wouldn't follow up with her appointments. She would mention how she wanted to see Thomas, but I would tell her that it was written in our agreement that I was to hear from her counselor before she was to have Thomas for a weekend. Fuck! I too just wanted some peace of mind.

> Kacey called at 2:50 a.m. I wasn't home. Her message was for me to call her. I don't know... Maybe if I procrastinate long enough, I will figure it out. I know I need more counseling. I have to dig up this root inside of me. Co-D(codependency)—If I had everything I ever wanted, I would question why I had it and why I wanted it. (JE, December 17, Sunday)
>
> Monday. Called Kacey back. Kacey was too pissed off to talk, said she'd call. I'm reading *Surviving Schizophrenia*. They're comparing it to manic depression. How strange it is to sit here knowing how bad-off someone is (Kacey), how serious the effects are (suicide), how easy it can be to recover (medication), and how hard it is to convince the people that can help (Kacey's parents). THAT is insanity. Oh, but wait. I am codependent. It is wrong to care or to worry about others. Mind your own. Serenity prayer? I'm praying for courage. No sympathy, till commitment. (Kacey) Repeat. (JE, December 18)
>
> Merry Christmas. Kacey called last night. She was crying off and on throughout our conversation. She was asking about our past. If I would have loved her had I not had a problem? Told her that I never would have gotten to know her if I didn't. She brought up how I was gone a lot—not just physically, but emotionally. I agreed.

Anytime I would bring up the thing about her getting help? Silence. She said she was getting a car and coming to see Thomas. I didn't have the heart to say no, but I didn't say yes either. I have to push her away and hope that she gets help, even though I still care for her. Tough love? No presents from Kacey for Thomas. Had my first dream about Kale. Okay. (JE, December 25)

Steve

(This is by far the most challenging task I've experienced while explaining these truths. There is no level of sensitivity that can be reached within my choice of words in order to safeguard and protect the feelings of those I care about as I still think of the Taylors as family. I simply have to continue to tell the truth.)

On New Year's Eve, Tanya and I asked Steve to accompany us to celebrate the New Year at a bar that a friend of ours had recently purchased. Steve politely declined our offer, so we went on without him. Tanya and I were having a fairly good time as I had rarely let her out of my sight in the past couple of months. At about 1:00 a.m., someone came into the bar and told Tanya that a police officer wanted to speak to her outside. She became frightened immediately and grabbed me as we quickly rushed out the door. The officer informed us that Steve had just committed suicide at his mother's home. He told us that Joan was at another officer's home near there and that we were to go there immediately. A few of our friends gathered us and drove us there.

If this is war, my enemy has just dropped the bomb. I surrender.

The details surrounding Steve's death are similar to Kale's, and I have no desire to share them. I already fear that I have become desensitized by reviewing this many times. I am desperately searching for the middle ground between telling the truth and remaining sensitive as I have kept Joan and Tanya in my thoughts at all times. I shared

Kale's details because I knew him well and I know he wouldn't mind. But I am unwilling to tell all of Steve's. I will let my edited journal write the rest.

> Steve killed himself on New Year's Eve! Details I'll never forget so I don't need to write them down. Schizophrenia. I don't know how much I'm supposed to dwell on this. Be Here Now (Was to be the title before I learned of the pre-existence of this book). Kacey, Kale, Steve. It's become my life. It's all I have on my mind. You cannot change your life unless you change your mind. Should you? Can You? Am I in denial or am I actually happy that Steve isn't in pain. What about Tanya and Joan? It can't hurt to learn more about schizophrenia. (AJE, January 3, 1996)
>
> (Steve would leave a note with Psalm 23. He said he would be with Daniel and Kale. He asked his family for forgiveness. He would also mention his love for his family and his admittance to feeling crazy.)
>
> A couple of our friends (Kale's, Steve's, mine) were at my apartment today. I learned a little more about Steve, except for the fact that our friend's minds cannot go where mine is. I told them some more about Kale. They can't add to it, or respond. I don't even know if they get it. (AJE, January 5, Friday)
>
> Tanya and her daughter went back to Joan's (were staying with me). Tanya worked today. She gave me Steve's journal—amazing. He shows constant suspicion. He was constantly talking about work, saying things like "I'm being set up, they want me to quit, and they're talking about firing me or kicking my ass or both." At the end of some of his entries, he would talk about God: "Don't exchange evil for evil, God help us all."

Etc. It didn't help matters that Kale felt the same way about his coworkers.

On January 28, 1995, Steve wrote: "Kale hit the boss today and was fired before noon. Kale thinks that a couple of coworkers tried to kill him. He said that if he starts acting crazy, to shoot him." The coworkers must be the two that Kale was talking about, but told me he couldn't say who they were for my own protection. Steve's last journal entry was dated October 11, 1995. His paranoia was increasing every day. Kale and Steve don't fear anyone, anymore. Not even themselves. (AJE, January 9, 1996)

Thomas is with Kacey's parents. Called and couldn't find Kacey. She had better not be where I think she is. (Due to missed appointments, she's currently not allowed unsupervised visits.) Was out last night. Talked to an old friend who knew Kale and Steve fairly well. He thinks they took the easy way out. Easy? I felt like smacking him. Just another reason to write and open these ignorant minds. Talked to my friend about the computer (to write). She is backing me with the money. She said it was okay as long as I promised to finish the book. Talked to Dan in California. He had been through Steve's camper. He heard a taped conversation (in which Steve himself recorded) that Steve had with the better business bureau. (Steve had called them about harassment at work.) Dan also said that when he went to get Steve's pickup at the airport, all the wires had been cut. (We assumed that Steve had cut them.) The security people at the airport knew Steve. He had confided in some of them. Asking them to stay by him because he felt that someone was after him. They said that he stood in one spot for

six hours. Sad. What the hell was he scared of?
Schizophrenia, to me, is like (thought) cancer of
the brain. (AJE, January 14, 1996, Sunday)

The discussion of schizophrenia continued in Wikipedia:

Genetics and early environment, as well as psychological and social processes, appear to be
important contributory factors. Some recre-
ational drugs appear to cause or worsen symptoms. The many possible combinations of symptoms have triggered debate about whether the
diagnosis represents a single disorder or a number
of separate symptoms...

Symptoms begin typically in young adult-
hood, and about 0.3–0.7% of people are affected
during their lifetime. In 2013, there was estimated to be 23.6 million cases globally. The disorder is thought to mainly affect the ability to
think, but it also usually contributes to chronic
problems with behavior and emotion. People
with schizophrenia are likely to have additional
conditions, including major depression and anxiety disorders; the lifetime occurrence of substance
use disorder is almost 50%. Social problems, such
as long-term unemployment, poverty, and home-
lessness are common. The average life expectancy
of people with the disorder is ten to twenty five
years less than the average life expectancy. This is
the result of increased physical health problems
and a higher suicide rate (about 5%). In 2013
an estimated 16,000 people died from behavior
related-to or caused by schizophrenia...

About 30–50% of people with schizophre-
nia fail to accept that they have an illness or their
recommended treatment. Treatment may have
some effect on insight.

Hello to Love

Death happens when you least expect it, death
　　happens when you do.
Like the rain that falls upon you; Inevitable and
　　true.
And as if they were never here, you say good-bye
　　to whom you hold dear.
And you put to rest another, and you hurt as if
　　your brother.
But with the passing of this day, those left we
　　always say,
'With He who lives above, good-bye to pain,
　　hello to love.'

(1996)

CHAPTER 18

Hindsight

To the living we owe respect, but to
the dead we owe only truth.

—Voltaire

(The following is my personal philosophy and my unprofessional opinion of how these events came to be, all of which may or may not reflect the assessment of the Taylor family. This is strictly my personal opinion and my philosophical views.)

Within the following months after Steve's death, I would come to learn that it was highly probable that Kale and Steve had been using meth in their recent past. It was likely called crystal or crank at that time and was often described, at least to me, as merely laced weed. Kale obviously never divulged any of this information about these drugs in our conversations as he knew I wouldn't approve. He likely saw no connection between drugs and his current condition. And at the time, I didn't think to ask more about it. I didn't begin my true concern for mental illnesses or their causes until Amanda introduced it to me sometime in the late fall of '94. Not knowing what I could've actually done with this information, I do regret not asking the right questions.

> Meth. Methamphetamine is a potent central nervous system stimulant of the phenethylamine and amphetamine classes that is used as a recreational drug and, rarely, to treat ADHD and

obesity … recreationally, meth is used to increase
sexual desire, lift the mood, and increase energy.
(Wikipedia)

I now understand that meth use can cause extreme paranoia,
possibly to the level of schizophrenia, in people who have had absolutely no genetic history of this mental illness in their family. I
learned that these people who do not have the family history have
a far better chance for recovery when they stop using. But Kale and
Steve were already highly vulnerable. Although preexisting, I believe
they activated their genetically inherited illness with this drug. Kale
and Steve's grandmother who lived with them in their teenage years
was said to be schizophrenic. Would their genetically inherited illness
have remained inactive? Could they have avoided active schizophrenia
by avoiding meth? That is the question we'll never be able to answer.
But with a history of schizophrenia already in their background, their
bloodline, there seemed to be a far less chance of recovering even
after they stopped using. Kale did everything that the doctors asked
of him, and I was in his presence long enough during his time home
from California, July '95, to know that he was no longer using, but
the damage was clearly done. This is what meth can do to you.

Although Kale would get on the wagon many times in his past,
more often than me anyway, he would often admit that he was likely
an alcoholic; something that definitely ran in his father's side of the
family. If I asked him why he was having a beer in the morning, he'd
casually reply, "Well, it isn't like I wasn't gonna drink today." As far
as Kale's recent depression, I understood his discontent to originate
from his thoughts of his brother. Although we rarely spoke of Daniel,
anyone who walks around feeling responsible for the death of a sibling is sure to develop some level of depression. But for a while, I
truly believed he had forgiven himself.

Once being concerned with a mutual friend several years back,
Kale and I discussed our friend's current state of mind. Every time
we saw him in a bar, this friend would make a reference to losing
someone many years ago.

"Why does he keep bringing up his sad past if it makes him feel
like shit?" I asked.

Kale answered, "I don't think he's thinkin' bout the past. Naw, he's likely just fuckin' depressed. He brings up the past cause he's tryin' to justify why he feels like shit all the time."

As many of us do, Kale once had the correct insight toward other's issues. But due to his current state of mind, he could no longer manage to apply this theory to his own life.

A few years after my friends' deaths (late '90s), I would accidentally snort crank. I say accidentally because it was not a conscious decision. I most likely had yet to completely comprehend the real connection between Kale's and Steve's past disorders to meth use. I didn't feel the need to inform myself about recent drugs as I rarely did anything other than smoke weed. Late one night, while in a drunken stupor, too far gone to have awareness of danger, a friend handed me a pocket rocket (nose inhaler). Possibly thinking it was cocaine, only after my second or third hit did I inquire about what it was. Oblivious to any danger, I unconcernedly asked, "So what does that mean to me?"

"About three days..." he comically replied as he informed me it was crank. I couldn't blame him for his offering. I'd never given him the impression I was against doing anything. And crank, I then considered crank to just be a form of speed. I took this information lightly because back in '91, I was occasionally taking mini thins, which were a form of a diet/energy pill that you could buy at any gas station. A lot of us did just to get through work when hungover. It was just a couple of steps above the average energy drink now. I didn't associate this to speed, crank, or meth, and even if I did, I don't think it would've swayed me at the time. And I don't know now if these drugs should be directly associated. You'd have to ask a chemist or a drug addict. I had literally no knowledge of meth then and still don't know if that's precisely what I consumed. I just remember being very high for quite a long time. I have never done it since. My point is, it's just that easy to do while drunk and unaware of your current surroundings. How Kale and Steve came across meth will forever be a mystery, but in my opinion, it was also likely not a conscientious decision. If the facts about the consequences of doing meth were as well-known then as they are now, I highly doubt they would've taken the chance.

I am very much aware of the fact that I wrote rather casually about the comedic side of my and Kale's drug and alcohol use, and I feel the need to clarify. If I had any inkling twenty-five years ago that such a lifestyle could lead to such tragic events, I would've obviously tried to do things differently. I chose to write the way I did in honor of authenticity and truth. And out of respect for my former self, chose to leave it through the editing process. There was just no other way to share this story. I feel it is much more important to be candid and honest than to be considerate—that's never gotten me anywhere. And I believe the truth about such matters educates more than formality ever will.

So in the fifteen years that Kale and I knew each other, although we drank together often, we smoked pot occasionally, we did cocaine together one time, we did Valium (sleeping pill) together one time, and we did acid together one time. I don't know Steve's drug history. I know Steve and I had never done anything other than pot together. And I was truly shocked to hear he'd likely been using meth. It just didn't seem to be in his character. As far as Kale's and my drug use is concerned and although we almost never experimented together, it is still debatable whether we were running from pain or simply in pursuit of pleasure. But whether you are aware of it or not, when you are sick most of the time, all you'll seek is pleasure. We were young. And when you're young, whether you are aware you of it or not, you are influenced by your friends. But I feel it is very important that you understand this: I was never pressured to do any of these drugs by Kale, and never did I pressure him—quite the opposite. I can remember Kale condemning me at times, warning me to be careful as he once considered pot to be the door to the house of drugs. I blame our ignorance on our youth and our individual chemical imbalances, not concussions, not our upbringing, not our childhood, but our own individual inherent genetic makeup. And if our problems require both cognitive therapy and a chemical resolution, isn't it most likely that it was always a chemical problem?

Although I blame schizophrenia for the deaths of my friends, depression was likely a daily issue in their previous years. What we rarely acknowledge is how depression is connected to drug use. I don't believe any mental illness goes without depression. Also considering myself, it's likely why we try any drug in the first place, unconsciously self-medicating. If you haven't yet decided to value yourself due to your upbringing or your chemical imbalance, if you do not fear the possible outcome of your future health, it's safe to assume you already have depression. Most of my experimentation was done spontaneously or while already under the influence of alcohol. Example– I don't think anyone wakes up in the morning and consciously says to himself, "I should try heroin today."

So do I believe depression can cause drug abuse? Yes. Do I believe drug abuse can cause depression? Yes. The same can happen with alcohol. Yet doctors now intentionally use marijuana and similar natural drugs to remedy depression and anxiety, among many other ailments. Go figure. They obviously seem to be seeking the proper balance. And it shouldn't be questioned. I recommend you use whatever your doctor prescribes as you cautiously remember that what can cure you can also make you ill.

Depression seems to accompany any mental illness whether we are conscious of it or not. Just the acknowledgment and recognition of any mental illness is sure to bring about depression if it didn't already exist; to become fully aware of one's state of mind, and then consider oneself crazy, will likely cause you to bring to life your negative internal dialogue, all unfairly due to the stigma surrounding this illness. And much in the same way we are all more susceptible to colds and flu, my inherited depression is often brought on by lack of sleep, hangovers, stress—the wearing down of my defenses. But I know now what is real and what isn't. When my depression arrives, no matter what twisted ideas and doubts enter my mind, I remind myself that this does not last, that this is a state of mind that, although it will reoccur, it is not me. And if it becomes more than I can handle, there is absolutely nothing wrong with walking into the doctor's office, sitting down, and saying, "I have depression. I need medication." (No further discussion needs to take place).

To put it simply, if you are depressed and in fear of the challenge to be well, know this: you can go to a doctor today, be prescribed an antidepressant, and within as soon as two weeks, your suicidal thoughts may disappear. That is the closest thing to a miracle. They likely cannot cure you, but living life without depression even temporarily will give you the necessary inspiration to survive it in the future. If these accumulative negative thoughts do arrive again in the future, go back. You wouldn't try to heal yourself, by yourself, of any other life-threatening illness. Why would depression be any different? Choose your own recovery path, but be true to yourself and follow it.

Although I have throughout this book, it's truly not fair to compare myself to both Kale and Steve. My childhood was different. My inherited chemical imbalance is different. If one considers schizophrenia to be the Niagara Falls of mental illnesses, my depression is now just a leaking faucet. But I do not take it lightly. And I can't count the hours in the past that I've envisioned my own demise. Believing I was the only one capable of raising my son first caused the realization that I simply cannot die. I don't have a choice. I have to get better. No matter what happens in the future, my child needs me. Because although I may have been wrong at the time, I felt I was truly all he had. I may be sick, but I can fake it long enough to take care of my son. I can find a way to live with depression if it means I have a chance to help him live without it.

As far as Kacey and I are concerned, when I look back, I may have been associating schizophrenia and manic depression as one in the same. Kacey has likely never experienced any form of psychosis (only she would know). I thought I had reasons to fear her running away with Thomas or possibly forgetting him somewhere, but I was likely falling into the stereotype that surrounds a mental illness. We would continue with our battle of wills for a few years. It became monotonous and luckily, stayed out the courtroom. I have no idea if she continued with medication. Every year Thomas grew older, my anxiety would lessen. I would ultimately mind my own business. I only regret the time I spent thinking of her when I should have been focused on those who truly wanted help, including myself. Years later, she would remarry and continue with her education eventually. Thomas would even come to live with her throughout much of his childhood. When he was old enough to make his own decision, he chose to live with me.

Although I assume she still hates me, I want to apologize to her for having shared much of our past with you. She's not likely to change her opinion of me upon reading this even though this was almost twenty years ago and I knew her for only three short years of her life. We were both very young and foolish. I regret that my attempts to help her long ago were only perceived as a means to control as she long believed she was still the center of my attention. "She's so vain. She probably thinks this book is about her." There was a time when she would laugh with me at that statement. I hope she still can.

Although I've sat in judgment of Kacey, Kale, and Steve, this book does not define them. Trust that there is much more to them than my story reveals. In my honest attempt to help others, I exposed what I believe to be all our issues involving only the psychological world. This is just my feeble storybook-psychologist insight into a few years of our lives together.

"Self-expression heals the wounded heart" (Anne Bancroft).

I truly had no idea where I was headed when I began writing. I am just as surprised as you to find out where it would lead. So to reiterate about my own personal journey of self discovery: psychology would tell me that I didn't receive enough hugs as a child, psychiatry tells me that I have a chemical imbalance that requires medication, religion would tell me to have more faith, and my philosophy tells me that I am just different from most, but still not alone with my thoughts of this illness. All or none of which may be true (my search continues). But I now understand myself to be someone who discovered many things during the course of honoring his late friends and most importantly, someone who found reason and direction in respect of the truth in order to move forward with the way I am.

I also want to apologize again to everyone I so freely chose to involve. That just because I've decided to expose my personal life, I shouldn't have the audacity to assume those I've involved will be in agreement. If this is the case, I'm truly sorry. This was written strictly from my perception of the truth, and I can only hope that they too view this not as an exploitation of their lives, but as a beneficial homage to those I have loved and learned from. I can only hope I have shown enough respect in that regard.

"Anyone who ever gave you confidence, you
owe them a lot" (Truman Capote).

I have had trouble determining the difference between confidence and arrogance as I can't recall truly being either one. I do feel it is somewhat of an act of arrogance just to write a book, believing that what I have to say is so important that you need to hear it. And although I have been honest, I still struggle to find the confidence to tell the truth in daily conversations. (Not afraid to, but I'm much too deep to be understood. I don't lie, I just withhold most thoughts.) I have also struggled to write confidently without offending for fear of sounding flippant. I'm still learning that confidence doesn't come from others. It truly comes from within. And it is in the act of being true to yourself that one can deter depression, anxiety, and the fear of judgment. It is when you doubt who you are that leads you susceptible to following the wrong path. To stand up for yourself in the face of peer pressure and bad advice is where you'll find peace within yourself. This affirmation is truly because of my friendship with Kale. I recall his abrasive advice to similar dilemmas when I would hesitate to share my thoughts with others: "Fuck 'em. Who are they to judge you? Speak from the heart and tell the truth." They will always know where you stand. My confidence to write this book came from this advice.

Kale has the words "Stop judging and start loving" on his tombstone. I'm aware that discernment is an inherent trait and necessary for survival, but judgment is not. My goal in the beginning was to remove wrongful judgment—judgment of my friends, judgment of those with mental illnesses, and judgment of me. And also to remove any possible conspiracy theories that may still roam the thoughts of those who knew my friends and still question what it was that happened to them. It would seem that our minds would rather believe in some conspiracy theory than to believe in no theory at all. So again, something did happen to Kale and Steve in California: they tampered with meth and opened up a part of their mind that made their silent negative thoughts and imagined delusions become real. A part of the mind that possibly exists in everyone, yet most of us are fortunate enough to have never explored. And if I can't change your judgments of them or your judgment of me, then maybe I can remove your own fear of being judged. We tend to walk around with secrets, and our secrets make us sick. When you don't fear the judgment from others, you don't fear telling your secrets. And revealing your secrets to the right people will help you to not feel so alone in your thoughts. Maybe I can convey the message that Kale taught me, as this book was supposed to be just about him: that being different is not something to hide; it's something to be proud of. He didn't fear judgment from strangers like I did. It's why I was drawn to him in the beginning. I don't think he feared judgment from anyone outside of his family. I just think he hated how critical and judgmental most people are. And he had the right. Although he was quick to make a judgment about physically defending himself or a friend during a confrontation, I almost never heard him criticizing anyone behind their back, just like the rest of his family. Kale understood that there is an untold story behind the eyes of everyone.

I do fear the repercussions from my second family as Joan can still be intimidating. I don't want them to think inversely of me. I believe that although I still feel close to them, we don't see one another nearly as often. I feel I may have been a reminder to them, not a sad reminder of the boys, but I likely remind them of the fragility of sanity—they know me well enough to have often worried about my mental health. And for a while, I may have kept my distance for the same reason. I want them to know that I'm okay.

I once asked Joan's advice on how to live consistently positive. I was told to put more of myself into my positive hobbies, whether that is fishing, hunting, motorcycles, or writing—to stay busy with what I love to do. As that is truly who you are and how you will be remembered. Well, this book is the result of one of my hobbies. I can only hope Joan appreciates it.

"Death makes angels of all; gives us wings where we once had shoulders smooth as ravens claws" (Jim Morrison).

My friends left our small community with everlasting memories. As recently as last spring, I would unintentionally run into Daniel's old high school girlfriend from 1983 at our local bar. I rarely see her; she's almost never in a bar. She is married with adult children and lives locally. I was a few beers into the night, so I tend to ask only the important questions. Before I mentioned that I'm writing a book about our late friends, I inquired about her time with Daniel. She told me that Daniel's birthday was just a few weeks ago. That she thought of him often. We reminisced. Several minutes later, I asked her, "How do you know you loved him?"

With a tear now in her eye, she solemnly replied, "It was the way he said my name."

What Jim Morrison was likely trying to tell us in his poem is that when you die young, your removal from our lives tends to elevate everything positive that you've done thus far. It seems one must die to become legend. But the price of receiving the amount of love and praise offered at one's own funeral should remain a price that no one is willing to pay. What good is the praise if you're not here to receive it? To view this objectively, my friends just didn't live long enough to disappoint, not long enough for me to ever think less of them.

I have elevated Kale, Daniel, and Steve to the degree of being more than human. Dealing with death will do this. But my gratitude for my time shared with them is real. We write about those who we perceive as worthy. We don't remember those for their kindness, generosity, or their love, we remember them for how they made us feel. And just as important, for remaining true to themselves. Right or wrong, it is men of conviction who will always be immortalized.

I could go on, but I believe I've held your attention long enough. I'm sorry I couldn't give you a happier ending. That's the thing about truth: it doesn't seem to care about your feelings. It also has no motive, and that's why I trust it enough to tell it.

Thanks for reading. I've come to learn that seasonal affective disorder is such a thing as it is likely what ails me. Everything affects our state of mind, from alcohol and drugs to something as simple as caffeine, diet, sleep, and yes, sunlight; some of the things you can sometimes control. The key is to try to be less sensitive and reactive to all substances. This includes the opinions from others while trying to remain true to yourself. Find out what it is that alters your perception of yourself. Not in the neurotic way I've done in the past, but in a simple act of being aware of what causes your own discomfort. And if you need professional help, go see a doctor. Fuck the stigma! You are just trying to survive. We all are.

Kale and I are parked on a gravel road, sitting in his car, enjoying a cigarette. When and where are irrelevant. We're leaning back admiring the stars through our open windows. There is a 12-pack between us. It was a good talk.

I tell Kale, "I do want to be a writer someday. I want to tell your story."

Without looking away from the night sky, he replies, "Do it. You gonna tell the truth?"

"Yeah."

"How much truth?" he asks.

"All of it," I answer.

He pauses. Still gazing at the stars, he exhales his smoke. "Well…, that's the question, Johnny … How much truth is there?"

This open-ended question would become part of my lifetime quest and ultimately lead to aiding me in my personal battle with depression. I have since discovered many truths; many powerful truths and philosophies that are very controversial. And due to the time required to share them, and out of respect for those involved in this story, I have chosen to leave them out of this book. (The next one is currently in progress.)

I still miss my friend, Kale. I miss all past personal relationships. I miss anyone who ever knew me well enough to exchange an unspoken, mutually understood look from across a crowded room. Nothing gives me more comfort and positive reinforcement on a daily basis than having someone you love understand you. And that is what I miss the most.

Thanks to the Taylor family and everyone who believed this possible.

> "Think where man's glory most begins and ends,
>   and say my glory was I had such friends."
>
> —William Butler Yeats

Justice

There are no words, yet I still try, to define the days since time passed you by.

The days sure seem longer than they once were and no one holds my attention, so I think of her.

I've looked to replace you, to pass time while I'm here.

They fall short of your memory and it's this that they fear.

I've been working on something that I hope makes you proud.

It's speaks of the truth and it's going to be loud.

It's the story of three brothers, a story of love, about your time here on earth and your journey above.

I hope you forgive me if it seems out of line,

But our friendships were important as I remember these times.

When you offered yourself and what you believed. So I'd be proud of who I am and cease to deceive.

So let the truth be revealed when I open their minds. And ask them to acknowledge their own troubled times. I hope to leave them at peace, although I've opened the door to take a look at themselves and see something more.

So if they close this book and look up to the sky,

Then I've given you justice... for being alive.

And may they finally put to rest their judgments and doubt, and be glad this book has left their lives out.

Justice...

(1996)

Journal 9/10/2016 Hello again! Didn't want to leave without saying good-bye. Editing has taken longer than I thought due to my damn day job and a few bouts with depression. It seems nothing is ever good enough when your mind is not in the right place. I'm still working on that. I've also started on the next book. Not even gonna guess when that will get done.

My son is well. Tobi is fine. The motorcycles are all okay. I have to return to my day job again for a while. I look forward to telling you more. Thanks for reading. ttyl.

ABOUT THE AUTHOR

John D. Day has been declared a 'storybook psychologist' and was once labeled as 'Johnny-with-the-news' by his best friend. After years of studying human behavior from a front row seat, he decided to share the story of his past relationships and some of the lessons involved. Although he has yet to declare victory over his own battle with depression, he continues to write during his seasonal time off in the upper Midwest.

Caroline,

Thanks for being a great host & becoming my friend. My friends are very important to me — as you will read. Keep in touch, I will be back to enjoy more motoX & your company! Go ELI! Thanks.

John D Day

CPSIA information can be obtained
at www.ICGtesting.com
Printed in the USA
FSOW02n0426240118
43609FS

9 781640 271418